Successful Prevention Programs for Children and Adolescents

Issues in Clinical Child Psychology

Series Editors: **Michael C. Roberts,** *University of Kansas–Lawrence, Kansas*
Lizette Peterson, *University of Missouri–Columbia, Missouri*

BEHAVIORAL ASPECTS OF PEDIATRIC BURNS
Edited by Kenneth J. Tarnowski

CHILDREN AND DISASTERS
Edited by Conway F. Saylor

CONSULTING WITH PEDIATRICIANS: Psychological Perspectives
Dennis Drotar

HANDBOOK OF ADOLESCENT HEALTH RISK BEHAVIOR
Edited by Ralph J. DiClemente, William B. Hansen, and Lynn E. Ponton

HANDBOOK OF CHILD BEHAVIOR THERAPY
Edited by T. Steuart Watson and Frank M. Gresham

HANDBOOK OF CHILDREN'S COPING:
Linking Theory and Intervention
Edited by Sharlene A. Wolchik and Irwin N. Sandler

HANDBOOK OF DEPRESSION IN CHILDREN AND ADOLESCENTS
Edited by William M. Reynolds and Hugh F. Johnston

INTERNATIONAL HANDBOOK OF PHOBIC AND ANXIETY
DISORDERS IN CHILDREN AND ADOLESCENTS
Edited by Thomas H. Ollendick, Neville J. King, and William Yule

MENTAL HEALTH INTERVENTIONS WITH PRESCHOOL CHILDREN
Robert D. Lyman and Toni L. Hembree-Kigin

SCHOOL CONSULTATION: Conceptual and Empirical Bases of Practice
William P. Erchul and Brian K. Martens

SUCCESSFUL PREVENTION PROGRAMS FOR CHILDREN
AND ADOLESCENTS
Joseph A. Durlak

Successful Prevention Programs for Children and Adolescents

Joseph A. Durlak

Loyola University Chicago
Chicago, Illinois

Plenum Press • New York and London

AHE 9474

Library of Congress Cataloging-in-Publication Data

Durlak, Joseph A.
   Successful prevention programs for children and adolescents /
Joseph A. Durlak.
       p.   cm. -- (Issues in clinical child psychology)
   Includes bibliographical references and index.
   ISBN 0-306-45645-1
   1. Child psychopathology--Prevention. 2. Adolescent
psychopathology--Prevention.   I. Title. II. Series.
   RJ499.D86 1997
   618.92'8905--dc21
                                                                97-18250
                                                                CIP

ISBN 0-306-45645-1

© 1997 Plenum Press, New York
A Division of Plenum Publishing Corporation
233 Spring Street, New York, N. Y. 10013

http://www.plenum.com

10 9 8 7 6 5 4 3 2 1

Preface

"An ounce of prevention is worth a pound of cure." "A stitch in time saves nine." When it comes to child and adolescent problems, are these phrases meaningless clichés? Is it really worthwhile to spend valuable time and effort attempting prevention when so many of our young people experience adjustment problems and urgently need attention? Are prevention programs effective? What type of problems can be prevented? Are there common elements or strategies that emerge among effective interventions? These are the questions addressed in this book.

Prevention is a multidisciplinary constellation of approaches directed at the prevention of disease and other types of negative outcomes and the promotion of health or other positive outcomes. Prevention works; that is, many well-done programs have significantly improved young people's subsequent adjustment, reduced future problems, or achieved both of these outcomes. Several programs have had dramatic effects. For instance, studies described in the following pages indicate that it is possible to reduce the future rate of clinical depression by 56%, serious acting-out behaviors by 50%, school vandalism by 79%, grade retentions by 33%, teenage pregnancies by 40%, and low-birth-weight infants by 42%. It is also possible to increase high school graduation rates by 24%, the proportion of children with positive mental health by 50%, and to double, triple, or quadruple the frequency of young people's healthy practices. In some cases, prevention has literally saved lives by reducing alcohol-related traffic fatalities by 26%, deaths due to falls by 35%, and fatal poisonings in young children by 75%.

Readers are likely to be pleasantly surprised, perhaps shocked, to learn of the success of so many prevention programs. For many years, rhetoric abounded regarding the value of prevention, but there were few solid scientific demonstrations of prevention effectiveness. In other words, people talked a lot about prevention, but did not practice it. That was then and this is now. There has been an explosion of research in prevention within the past 20 years, and there are now over 1200 published prevention outcome studies.

Thoughtfulness, patience, and systematic effort are required to mount effective prevention programs, and not every intervention has been successful. Therefore, it is important to highlight empirically validated programs. Such information is particularly important from a policy perspective because there are many current programs identified as prevention programs whose impact is unknown. These programs may not be very effective and can produce a false impression of what prevention is and what it can accomplish. Furthermore, it is irresponsible to waste valuable and limited resources such as time, money, and personnel on programs of questionable impact when there are better alternatives.

Therefore, I discuss exemplary programs throughout this book. I have selected representative programs in different areas that have been carefully conceptualized, conducted, and evaluated. I emphasize programs that are theory driven; that is, programs that rest on a theoretical and conceptual base, or, at the very least, are guided by previous empirical findings and attempt to test specific a priori hypotheses. When examining program design, I looked for studies that addressed matters of internal and external validity. Internal validity affects the confidence of any conclusions about a program's impact. External validity involves the degree to which results can be generalized, and so I highlight interventions that have been replicated one or more times, especially if independent investigators evaluated similar programs conducted across different populations and settings.

In terms of program evaluations, I looked for studies that used psychometrically adequate outcome measures and multiple measures, collected some follow-up data, and assessed changes in behavior or adjustment status. Prevention attempts to do something now to prevent later difficulties, so it is important to monitor program effects over time. Although several early preventive interventions attempted to change children's knowledge or attitudes, we now know that the critically important outcomes involve behavioral change. Have children's behaviors improved following intervention? Is academic performance enhanced? Does their health status change? Do they take fewer risks that would lessen the likelihood of negative consequences associated with driving, drinking, or having sex? I emphasize these types of outcomes when discussing the results of different programs.

Space limitation prohibits discussing every well-done investigation. Nevertheless, the programs that are described represent good working models for the design, implementation, and evaluation of preventive interventions. In general, I use a weight of evidence approach to reach conclusions in each specific area and for the field of prevention in general. In summary, this text presents a panoramic snapshot of current findings in prevention with an emphasis on the very best programs.

Hopefully, this book will encourage more students and professionals to become involved in prevention. Positive results from empirical studies will not automatically lead to more prevention, however. If prevention is as successful as current outcome data suggest, then it is appalling that most current efforts in medicine, mental health, education, and the social services are still directed at treating individuals with established problems instead of trying to prevent such outcomes in the first place. The full potential of prevention will not be realized until we understand and overcome the political, personal, and administrative barriers that impede prevention practices.

I have written this book for a wide audience that includes preventionists, service providers, and students from multiple disciplines. Covering multiple fields should be instructive. Those already active in prevention should be pleased to learn that many of the strategies used in their domain are also being applied successfully in other areas. This convergence across diverse areas increases confidence that prevention rests on sound scientific principles. Others wishing to learn what prevention is and how it is accomplished will encounter plenty of useful information. Prevention is a multidisciplinary science, and work in many different areas is discussed: mental and physical health, academics, child abuse, injuries, AIDS, pregnancy, and so on. As a result, this text is relevant to those in medicine and nursing, psychology, education, social work, social and child welfare, and family and policy studies.

I want to acknowledge several people who have influenced my work. Many undergraduate and graduate students over the years have assisted me in my research on prevention and community psychology. I want to express my appreciation to this group for their interest, enthusiasm, and support. I undertook the task of writing this book cautiously. First, I wrote a monograph for Alan Kazdin's *Developmental and Clinical Psychology and Psychiatry* series on school-based prevention programs (Durlak, 1995). His positive editorial reaction suggested that I had produced something of value and so I developed some confidence in my ability to undertake a larger project. Then Lizette Peterson and Mike Roberts, the co-editors of the *Issues in Clinical Child Psychology* series for Plenum, paid me the ultimate compliment of asking me to write this book. Both Mike and Lizette were extremely helpful and supportive throughout the project. They showered me with reprints and materials to get me started on areas in which they, not I, were the experts, such as injury prevention and pediatric psychology. They were also quick to review chapter and manuscript drafts and they kept praising my work. All authors should have such kind and helpful editors.

When I first met Mariclaire Cloutier at Plenum, I knew I was in good hands. She has waited patiently for this book and has marshalled it along during the publication process. Finally, my wife, Chris, has been a constant source of support and an invaluable editorial assistant.

JOSEPH A. DURLAK

Contents

1. Basic Concepts in Prevention 1

What Is Prevention? 1
    New Terminology for Prevention 1
Different Approaches to Prevention 2
    Selecting Target Populations 2
    Level of Intervention 3
Indicated Prevention 6
Multiple Goals of Prevention 6
Critical Questions in Prevention 7
Important Themes in Prevention 8
    Multiple Causality 9
    Risk and Protective Factors 10
    Health Promotion 12
    Developmental Pathways 13
    Systematic Skills Training 17
Brief History of Prevention 17
    Early History 17
    History of Prevention in Mental Health 18
    Current History of Prevention 20
    Current Research and Practice on Prevention 21
Plan of the Book 24
Summary 24

2. Prevention of Behavioral and Social Problems 27

Introduction 27
Primary Prevention Programs 28
    Person-Centered Programs 30

Mental Health Promotion 31
Transition Programs 32
Environment-Centered Programs 36
Indicated (Secondary) Prevention 42
    General Overview 42
    Screening Procedures 43
    The Legacy of the Primary Mental Health Project 44
    Brief Review of Indicated Prevention Programs 46
    Program Examples 48
    A Community-Based Study 51
Summary 52

3. **Prevention of Learning Problems** 55

Extent of Child Learning Problems 55
Factors Affecting Learning 56
Importance of Early Intervention 57
Early Childhood Programs 57
    The Legacy of Head Start 57
    Program Examples 59
    Elements of Successful Interventions 61
Interventions at the Elementary Level 63
    Tutoring 63
    Success for All 64
Indicated Prevention 65
    Characteristics of Effective Interventions 66
Classroom and School Factors 67
    Classroom Environments 67
    Effective Schools 68
    Making Schools More Effective 70
    Importance of Social Norms and Values 72
    Good Academic Performance as a Protective Factor 73
Summary 73

4. **Drug Prevention** 75

Introduction 75
Brief History of Drug Interventions 76
Successful Drug Prevention Programs 77
    Skills Training Programs 77
    Communitywide Programs 79
    Timing and Duration 83
    Program Generalization 84

Effective Program Elements 84
A Special Word about Smoking 84
Drug Use versus Misuse 85
Gap between Research and Practice 85
Summary 86

5. **Programs to Improve Physical Health** 87

Introduction 87
Programs for Pregnant Women and Young Children 88
Smoking during Pregnancy 88
Passive Smoking Programs 89
Other Interventions for Families with Young Children 91
Guidelines for Effective Early Health Intervention 94
Guideline 1: Target High-Risk Groups 95
Guideline 2: Consider Health in Broad Terms 95
Guideline 3: Emphasize Effective Service Delivery Practices 97
Programs for School-Age Children 98
Transformation of School-Based Health Education 98
Sex Education and AIDS and Pregnancy Prevention 106
Characteristics of Effective Programs 107
Representative Programs 108
Sexuality and AIDS 110
Pregnancy Prevention 111
Summary 113

6. **Injury Prevention** 115

Introduction 115
Additional Facts about Injury 116
Approaches to Injury Prevention 117
Environmental Interventions 118
Effects of Legislation 118
Child Car Safety Devices 119
Wearing of Bicycle Helmets 121
Prevention of Other Types of Injuries 122
Elements of Effective Community Programs 126
Individual Level Interventions 127
Training Children in Safety Behaviors 127
Latchkey Children 128
Interventions by Physicians 129
Summary 129

7. Child Maltreatment 131

Introduction 131
  Consequences of Maltreatment 131
Physical Abuse and Neglect 132
  Risk and Protective Factors 132
  Representative Programs 134
Prevention of Sexual Abuse 137
  Primary Prevention 137
  Indicated (Secondary) Prevention 139
Summary 140

8. Is Prevention Cost-Effective? 143

Introduction 143
Benefit–Cost Analyses of Prevention 144
  Example 1: Modest Outcomes Can Be Cost-Effective 147
  Examples 2 and 3: Need for Follow-up 147
  Example 4: Factors Interact to Determine Outcomes 148
  Example 5: Cost Analysis with an Explicit Policy Thrust 150
Cost-Effectiveness Analysis 150
  Time as a Program Cost 151
  Program Benefits 153
  Comparing Alternative Interventions 156
  A Caution 157
Summary 158

9. Importance of Policy 159

Introduction 159
  Overview of Policy Research 160
Effects of Specific Policies 160
  School Policies 160
  Taxation of Tobacco Products 161
  Taxation of Alcoholic Products 162
  Effects of Legislation 163
  Limiting Minors' Access to Cigarettes and Alcohol 167
  Barriers to Enforcement 170
  Drafting of Legislation 171
Influencing Policy 172
  Top-down Approaches 172
  Bottom-up Approaches 173
  Potential Problems 174

Need for a Stronger Policy on Prevention 175
Summary 175

10. Current Status and Future Directions 177

Introduction 177
Major Research Findings 177
    Prevention Works 177
    Prevention Has Practical Benefits 178
    An Important Qualification 180
Guidelines for Improving Programs 181
    Implications from Risk Research 181
    Emphasize Protective and Positive Factors 188
    Begin from a Sound Theoretical and Empirical Base 192
    Involve Parents as Much as Possible 192
    Abandon the Use of Information-Only Programs 192
    Compare Alternative Programs 193
    Adopt a Long-Term Perspective 193
    Be Flexible in Providing Services 193
    Pay Careful Attention to Program Implementation 194
    Expand Possible Sites for Prevention 195
    Use a Collaborative Approach 195
    Work with Community Coalitions 196
    Use Mass Media and Technology Effectively 197
    Combine Qualitative and Quantitative Approaches 198
    Offer More Comprehensive Interventions 198
The Future of Prevention 199
    Concluding Comments 200
Summary 201

Appendix A. Characteristics of Effective Skill Training
Programs 203

Appendix B. Helpful Resources on Prevention 205

References 213

Author Index 233

Subject Index 237

1

Basic Concepts in Prevention

WHAT IS PREVENTION?

Prevention is a multidisciplinary science that draws upon basic and applied research from at least 15 major disciplines: education, psychology, medicine, nursing, public health, sociology, political science, business, communications, law, criminal justice, social work, health education, engineering, and economics. In addition, some of the specialty areas of these disciplines that have made important contributions to prevention are early childhood education, community psychology, community nursing, pediatrics, epidemiology, social marketing, policy analysis, and community organization and development.

Many different frameworks and concepts have been used to describe prevention. Caplan (1964) described three types of prevention that differ in their purpose and timing: primary, secondary, and tertiary prevention. Primary prevention is an intervention for normal populations designed to prevent the future occurrence of problems. Secondary prevention is intervention for populations with early problems to forestall the development of more serious difficulties. Tertiary prevention aims to reduce the duration or consequences of established problems or disorders.

New Terminology for Prevention

Over time, tertiary prevention has become so confused with therapy or rehabilitation that most preventionists now emphasize that only interventions occurring before the onset of serious problems should be considered preventive interventions (Institute of Medicine, 1994). I adopt this philosophy and only consider primary and secondary pre-

vention programs, which are explained more completely in the following sections. The Institute of Medicine (1994) has suggested the use of
the terms, *selective preventive intervention* for a primary prevention
high-risk approach (see below) and *indicated preventive intervention* to
refer to all secondary prevention programs. The old and new terms for
primary and secondary prevention are used interchangeably throughout this text to remind readers of the new proposed terminology for
prevention.

DIFFERENT APPROACHES TO PRIMARY PREVENTION

There is no single approach that has been used in primary prevention. Although slightly different terms have been used, many agree that
current primary prevention programs differ in two major respects:
(1) the ways target populations are selected for intervention, and (2) the
level of intervention that is emphasized (Cowen, 1986; Price, 1986).
Figure 1.1 illustrates 15 distinctions that are possible depending on
which of three selection procedures and five levels of intervention are
emphasized.

Selecting Target Populations

One approach, called a population-wide or universal strategy, targets all in a designated population for intervention. Examples of universal strategies would be programs for all junior high school students, all
parents of first grade children, or all members of a geographically defined community. A second strategy, a high-risk approach (that is, selective preventive intervention), targets groups who are at risk for problems
but who are not yet demonstrating any difficulties. Because young children from low-income households are at higher risk for subsequent
academic problems than those from families at a higher socioeconomic
status, a high-risk strategy in primary prevention would target the former group for intervention. Children of depressed parents represent
other high-risk groups, because in general these children are more likely
to have more adjustment difficulties than children of nondepressed
parents.

The final selection strategy, the milestone or transition approach,
focuses on those children about to undergo critical life transitions or
stressful life events. The rationale for this approach is that certain life
tasks or events are particularly difficult or stressful and can produce

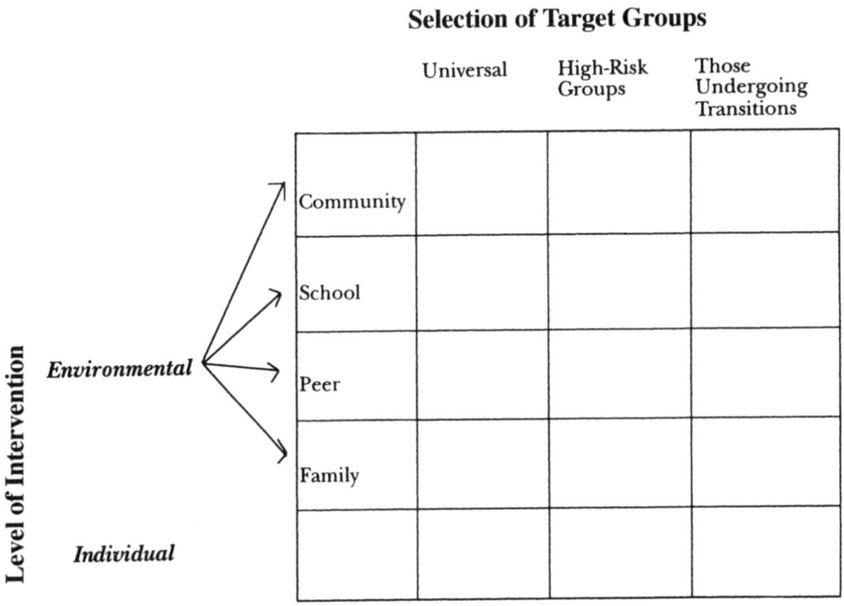

Selection of Target Groups

	Universal	High-Risk Groups	Those Undergoing Transitions
Community			
School			
Peer			
Family			

Environmental (Community, School, Peer, Family)

Individual

Level of Intervention

Figure 1.1. Conceptual overview of approaches to primary prevention.

lasting negative effects. Interventions are designed to help children negotiate these transitions effectively. Children changing schools, children of divorcing parents, and those about to experience medical and dental treatment could all be potential candidates for the milestone or transition approach to primary prevention.

Level of Intervention

The second major distinction in primary prevention involves the level of intervention, and there are five possibilities: a person-centered (or individual-level) approach and four levels of environment-centered programs. In the individual-level approach, change agents work directly with children or adolescents to prevent specific problems or to promote well-being, whereas environmental interventions attempt to change youth by changing their environment. Environmental interventions can occur at four different levels: the family, the peer group, the school (or other social organization), and the community. The five levels of intervention are depicted in the rows in Fig. 1.1.

Many environmental interventions stress ecological principles and are sometimes called ecological or systems-level interventions. There are several important elements of ecological theory (Bronfenbrenner, 1979; Sameroff, 1987). First, ecological theories stress that there are many social and organizational influences on behavior, and individual behavior should not be considered apart from their context. Although response contingencies influence behavior, so can values, norms, expectations, social policies, and the behaviors of others in a setting. Access to needed resources is another important influence. For example, Levine, Toro, and Perkins (1993) noted that federal law prohibiting local schools from expelling pregnant adolescents was probably the single-most important factor that increased graduation rates of pregnant adolescents since 1956. The federal law removed an important barrier in preventing pregnant teens from completing their high school education.

Second, ecological theories stress the importance of examining person–environmental interactions and acknowledging that some individuals will do better in one type of setting over another. Thus, determining the best person–environment fit for different individuals is crucial.

Third, an ecological approach examines bidirectional and transactional processes. In the former case, child behavior can affect adult behavior, just as the reverse is possible. A transactional perspective further extends these views by noting that bidirectional effects produce a new, evolving interactive sequence of interpersonal behaviors over time. For instance, a child's behavior affects the parent's behavior, which in turn affects the child's behavior. Transactional processes can produce a series of positive, mutually satisfying behaviors and events or a string of negative, aversive behaviors.

A good example of the latter is the discovery of coercive interactions occurring for many children who have serious behavioral problems. Basically, in a coercive interaction the participants learn to control each other's behavior by negative means. A child may begin the sequence by demanding something and then escalate his or her behavior until a full-blown tantrum is in progress. At the same time a parent's behavior is also escalating. Initially, a parent might ignore the child; but the child's continual pressure influences the parent who first said no to then yell or scold, and then perhaps to physically restrain or slap the child. Ultimately, however, the parent gives in to the child's demand. Both parties are being reinforced in this interaction: The child receives what was initially desired and the parent is reinforced because the child's aversive behavior has temporarily ceased. As a result, the coercive cycle will continue. Viewed from an ecological perspective, preventive interventions attempt to eliminate negative transactional processes or to initiate positive transactional processes that will enhance adjustment and prevent negative outcomes.

Most environmental interventions attempt to change the social aspects of the environment, that is, the behavior of people in settings. Changing the behavior of significant others in the child's environment (peers, parents, and teachers) is expected to lead to positive behavior change in the child. Attempts to change parental child-rearing practices are a prime example of family-level interventions. Other family-oriented programs seek to empower parents to become more effective advocates for their children, or provide social support to parents as they attempt to improve their own and their children's adjustment. The general idea is to improve the home environment and family system in order to foster child development.

Peer interventions are common in drug, physical health, and some mental health programs. Peer role models are used to help youth resist pressures to take drugs, improve nutrition and exercise patterns, and improve their social skills. Environmental interventions at the level of the school might consist of changes in school policies and curricula or teachers' management and organization of the classroom. Drafting legislation to fund new services, changing social norms to increase or decrease certain behaviors (e.g., smoking), developing communitywide interventions, mounting mass media campaigns, or taxing products such as alcohol or cigarettes are examples of approaches that might be taken at the community level.

Finally, a few environmental programs emphasize the physical environment. This is most apparent in the field of injury prevention when products are redesigned to be safer (e.g., potentially hazardous substances are sold in "child-resistant" packages) or when the physical environment is changed in some way (e.g., window guards are installed in high-rise apartments to prevent falls; see Chapter 6).

The different approaches depicted in Fig. 1.1 are not mutually exclusive, given that interventions at different levels can be combined. For instance, many environmental programs include an individual-level component, so the major distinction between person and environmental programs is whether the intervention attempts some modification of the social or physical environment. This distinction is important because of growing evidence in some areas of prevention that programs that are most successful over the long term intervene at one or more environmental levels. In other words, there may be limits to what can be accomplished if one's approach is restricted to the individual level of intervention.

As further examples of how multiple levels of interventions can be combined, some large-scale, community-oriented programs combine all five levels of intervention. These programs consist of components for children, parents, and teachers; mass media campaigns; and efforts to promote policy initiatives and new community services (Chapter 4 presents some examples). Finally, methods of selecting target groups can also be blended. A transition program may focus only on those at risk rather than all youth undergoing the transition (Jason et al., 1992; see Chapter 2). In summary, although there can be overlap in the level of intervention and identification of target groups used in prevention programs, the schema depicted in Fig. 1.1 is still useful for distinguishing among interventions.

INDICATED PREVENTION

Whereas primary prevention intervenes with healthy or normal individuals, indicated (secondary) prevention provides help to those who demonstrate early problems. Some systematic screening or case-finding approach is used to identify those in need of attention. For instance, all junior high school students may be screened using a psychological battery and only those with the highest levels of test anxiety receive treatment. The basic intent of secondary prevention is to prevent more serious dysfunction from occurring through early intervention; "to nip problems in the bud," so to speak. For the most part, this volume discusses primary rather than secondary prevention, but there are separate sections devoted to secondary prevention in Chapters 2, 3, and 7. Theoretically, the same five levels of intervention used in primary prevention can also be applied to secondary prevention. In practice, however, the majority of indicated prevention programs have been individual-level interventions.

MULTIPLE GOALS OF PREVENTION

Prevention can have four major goals: (1) to prevent new problems from appearing; (2) to prevent early, milder problems from becoming more serious; (3) to lessen the seriousness of any new problems that develop; and (4) to delay the onset of problems. The first two goals are the traditional ones associated with primary and secondary (indicated) prevention, but the latter two goals are also important. Intervening so that any new problems that appear are less serious is an important accomplishment. Milder problems are much less likely to have profound, long-term effects on adjustment. Finally, delaying the onset of problems is another worthy preventive goal. There are considerable data indicating that the earlier the problems appear, the more likely they are later to lead to more serious difficulties. This is so for early sexual activity and drug use, aggression and other forms of externalizing behavior, learning problems, and various unhealthy behaviors such as poor diet and nutrition, exercise patterns, and smoking (see Durlak, 1995; Hawkins, Catalano, & Miller, 1992; and Chapters 2–7, this volume). Therefore, interventions do not have to completely eliminate problems to be beneficial.

CRITICAL QUESTIONS IN PREVENTION

There are several critical questions confronting prevention, some of which are listed in Table 1.1. For instance, what is the best way to identify normal individuals who are at risk but who do not yet have any problems (that is, do selective primary prevention)? What is the best way to conceptualize and assess different features of the environment? What person–environment interactions and bidirectional and trans-

Table 1.1. Some Critical Questions
Facing Current Approaches to Prevention

Selecting target populations for intervention
 1. Under what circumstances are universal, high-risk, and transition approaches most effective?
 2. What is the best way to identify normal individuals who are at future risk, but who do not yet have any problems (i.e., mount selective prevention interventions)?
 3. For secondary (indicated) prevention, how can we identify in the most reliable and valid fashion those who are just beginning to show difficulties?
 4. How do transitions influence development?
 5. What helps youth master difficult life transitions?
 6. Can we determine who is at greater or lesser risk for different transitions?
Levels of intervention
 1. What level of intervention or what combination of levels is most effective?
 2. What is the best way to conceptualize and assess the environment?
 3. What person–environment, bidirectional, and transactional interactions are most important?
 4. How can we secure maximum participation of parents, teachers, peers, and community groups?

Note: Each of the above questions needs to be answered in reference to different goals, populations, and settings.

actional processes are most important in different circumstances and how can these be translated into effective interventions? How do transitions create problems for children and how can we help youth master difficult life transitions?

It is important to clarify how different levels of interventions can be used most effectively with different methods of selecting target populations, because there are trade-offs involved in these approaches. There is usually no stigma attached to participating in universal primary prevention programs because all in the population are targeted, but environmental interventions are often more difficult to conduct than individual-level interventions. For instance, it is usually easier to secure the participation of schoolchildren who are a captive group compared to involving most eligible parents, teachers, and various community groups in programs.

Furthermore, in universal interventions some will not benefit because they do not need the intervention in the first place; at the same time, universal programs cannot usually be very intensive or lengthy because of limited money or personnel. As a result, some in the target population might not benefit because they need a more intensive program. In effect, the program's resources may not be well spent. A high-risk approach might be preferable in primary prevention if there is an efficient way of determining risk and if the intervention is sufficiently powerful to help those at higher risk.

In terms of environmental interventions, it is reasonable to assume that systemic and organizational processes can reach more children and possibly produce enduring behavioral changes. For example, if effective new school policies and educational curricula can be instituted on a permanent basis, these changes will affect many students year after year. The drawback to these higher-order levels of change is that they can be much more difficult to achieve, and thus require much more time and effort than individual-level programs.

Current prevention programs reflect a creative mix of ideas in response to the above questions and dilemmas. Although many issues have yet to be resolved, research findings are beginning to indicate the value of different approaches. This information is highlighted in the following chapters whenever it is available.

IMPORTANT THEMES IN PREVENTION

There are five important themes in prevention that help in understanding the assumptions and strategies that guide many current interventions. These five themes relate to multiple causality, risk and protective factors, health promotion, developmental pathways, and the importance of systematic skill training. These themes are often combined in interventions because they are closely related to each other, but each merits separate discussion.

Multiple Causality

The view has been expressed that prevention cannot be very successful because the causes of most adjustment problems are unknown (Lamb & Zusman, 1979). In other words, how can we prevent something bad from happening if we do not know what causes it in the first place?[1] This perspective rests largely on a medical model that suggests there is a specific and unique cause for different outcomes.

In prevention, it is assumed that most outcomes are multiply determined. We will probably never discover a missing link or single causal agent for most problems or negative outcomes. Therefore, it is important to develop programs that can modify some of the factors that presumably influence development and then examine their short- and long-term effects. Careful inspection of the outcome data will determine whether research and practice are on the right path.

Longitudinal developmental research demonstrating the principles of divergent and convergent development and the presence of developmental discontinuities clearly supports the notion of multiple causality (Sameroff, 1987). These principles are illustrated in Fig. 1.2. The principle of divergent development stresses that the same starting point can be associated with different outcomes. Note that point B in Fig. 1.2 can lead to outcomes D, E, *or* F. The principle of convergent development is that the same final result can develop from different starting points. The same final good outcome, point D, can occur for those beginning at starting points A, B, *or* C. The same factors do not always lead to the same results because developmental discontinuities occur. Discontinuities refer to major breaks or shifts in the developmental process that lead to different outcomes (e.g., point C, poor initial adjustment, nevertheless can lead to a good final outcome, point D). In other words, the

[1]This same objection has never been seriously expressed with respect to psychotherapy. Clinical theories emphasize different and sometimes contradictory causes for various personal and social problems, but psychotherapists have not waited until these theories have been resolved before intervening to assist those in need of help. Furthermore, there is substantial evidence that psychotherapy is generally effective for both children and adolescents (Weisz, Weiss, Han, Granger, & Morton, 1995), indicating that behavior can be modified without knowing its initial cause.

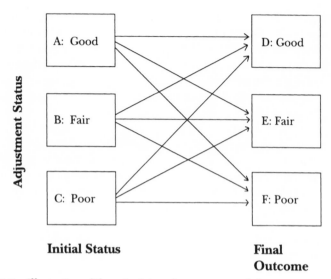

Figure 1.2. Illustration of the principles of convergent and divergent development.

developmental process is not perfectly linear. If it were, then all normal infants would become normal adults and all infants who have early physical or behavioral problems would eventually have later difficulties. We know this does not happen.

Risk and Protective Factors

Risk and protective factors have become important concepts in prevention for targeting different groups for intervention, deciding what to emphasize in the program, and evaluating outcomes. Risk and protective factors relate to the future likelihood of negative and positive outcomes, respectively. A risk factor increases the possibility of some negative outcome, while a protective factor either reduces the chances of a negative outcome or increases the chances of a positive outcome.[2]

At the individual level, risk can be a demographic characteristic (low-income level), a behavior (delinquent activity or unprotected sexual intercourse), or an inaccurate perception or piece of information (e.g., all forms of contraception are equally effective). At the family

[2]Adequate terminology is lacking in reference to positive health. For factors that increase the occurrence of positive outcomes, the term, *positive factor*, is probably more appropriate than protective factor, because the latter term implies avoidance of something negative, which is not the same thing as a decidedly positive outcome.

level, risk can refer to low maternal education, inconsistent discipline practices, or lack of warmth. At other levels, risk may include others who use drugs, the lack of social support, a school with poor levels of achievement, or a community policy that limits access to certain types of care. In other words, risk factors can be present at all levels, and some factors are more amenable to influence than others.

Risk research indicates that negative outcomes are not related to single factors but to a combination or accumulation of factors, and that risk factors seem to have multiplicative effects. For example, Rutter (1979) studied six risk factors related to child psychiatric disorders, such as maternal psychopathology, severe marital discord, and paternal criminality. There were no outcome differences between children exposed to none of the factors and those exposed to any one of the six, but those experiencing two or three risks were five times more likely and those experiencing four to six risks were 20 times more likely to have a clinical disorder.

Other studies contain similar findings. One report found that 11-year-old children exposed to eight or more of ten risk factors were six times more likely to have behavior problems than children exposed to zero or only one (Williams, Anderson, McGee, & Silva, 1990). Another study (Sameroff, Seifer, Zax, & Barocas, 1987) found that ten times more children experiencing seven or eight (out of a possible ten) risk factors were viewed as clinically disturbed than children exposed to less than two.

The presence of risk factors at multiple levels and their multiplicative effects have strong implications for prevention. The most successful programs are likely to be multilevel interventions that can reduce the multiple risks present at several levels.

Much more needs to be learned about risk and protective factors. There is no standardized approach in identifying and measuring risk, and usually different combinations of factors are related to different outcomes. Consistent with the principles of convergent and divergent development, many different risk factors can be related to the same outcome and the same risk factor can be associated with several different outcomes. This makes understanding the exact relationship between risk and outcome very difficult.

Moreover, risk and protective factors are currently much more useful in predicting outcomes for *populations* rather than for *individuals*. Groups with more risk factors have a higher probability of a negative outcome than those with fewer risks, but the ability to predict exactly who will have later problems is far from perfect. For instance, among the studies cited above, only 30% (Sameroff et al., 1987) or 40% (Williams et al., 1990) of those at the highest levels of risk had problems. Therefore, even at relatively high levels of risk, all individuals will not experience negative outcomes, perhaps because of the presence of unidentified protective factors.

In theory, the same principles hold for protective factors as for risk factors; that is, protective (positive) factors exist at multiple levels (individual, family, and so on), and the more protective factors that are present, the higher the likelihood of positive outcomes. Research has identified far more risk than protective factors, however, and the two are not simply the opposite of each other. For instance, aggression in childhood is a risk factor, but the lack of aggression is not a protective factor. The major protective factors that have been identified so far include a warm and supportive parent, availability of an effective social support system, and, to some extent, good interpersonal or social skills. Good academic performance may also serve as a protective factor. Rutter (1979) reported data showing that children with good reading skills were much less likely to have school behavior problems than children with poor reading skills. These results held for children coming from high-risk as well as low-risk homes. Another study (Zingraff, Leiter, Johnsen, & Myers, 1994) found a significant association between physical abuse and neglect and later delinquent activity, but this relationship was greatly reduced if children were performing well in school. Further evidence that good academic performance can be a protective factor is presented in Chapter 3.

Finally, identifying what factors produce risk or increase protection does not explain how these factors operate. What is it about social support that helps protect individuals? More information is needed to explain the developmental processes by which risk and protective factors operate to influence development.

Health Promotion

Health promotion has become an important element in prevention. The general idea behind health promotion is to increase the skills, strengths, or coping abilities of target groups; that is, to focus on positive aspects of health or adjustment. Health promotion is based on the rationale that children and adolescents with enhanced competencies and coping abilities should be able to attain personal goals more effectively and be better able to deal with stress and to master various developmental tasks. In effect, health promotion should lead to fewer future problems, because good health is a protective factor in children's lives.

A clinical example illustrates this point. Suppose that two young adults, Jim and Jack, enter therapy with the same level of depression and anxiety that affects both job performance and interpersonal relation-ships. Each client ends psychotherapy showing similar reductions in depression and anxiety, but there is a substantial difference between the two clients in their positive characteristics and skills. Compared to Jim, Jack feels much happier and has much more self-confidence. Jack has renewed energy for his job and has become assertive with his colleagues and boss so that he is no longer overburdened with unreasonable de-mands and deadlines. Furthermore, he is optimistic as he begins to date. He has developed a healthy sense of humor and has learned how to relax to reduce tension and stress when they occur. Which client has a better prognosis overall and what is the major difference between the two?

Although both clients are without major symptomatology at treat-ment termination, most would agree that prospects seem much brighter over the long run for Jack than for Jim because the former has better mental health. Jack now has some positive skills and qualities that not only appear to make him happier and more self-confident, but also will probably serve him well when he encounters future stress. Basically, the same argument can be made for preventive interventions that empha-size health promotion. Programs that reduce problems *and* increase competencies probably leave their participants at lower risk for future difficulties than those that only achieve the former outcome.

Although there is some debate over the value of health promotion (Institute of Medicine, 1994), many programs use health promotion activities to prevent maladjustment. For example, programs that have successfully prevented aggression and serious acting-out problems have trained children in self-control strategies and various social skills (Hawkins, Von Cleve, & Catalano, 1991). The strategy was to replace the child's customary antisocial behavior with prosocial forms of behavior.

Health deserves attention in its own right because it is not the opposite of illness or maladjustment. A person without a physical ill-ness or any symptoms is not necessarily one who is physically fit and healthy. As the above example of the two therapy clients, Jack and Jim, illustrates, someone who is no longer depressed is not necessarily happy, self-confident, or socially skilled. Therefore, some prevention-ists believe that one way to forestall future problems is promote well-ness (Cowen, 1994).

Developmental Pathways

Developmental pathways are basically roadmaps illustrating the course of adjustment and maladjustment over time. There can be differ-ent pathways for single behaviors and constellations of behaviors, for competencies and problems, and for different populations.

For instance, five major developmental pathways have been identified in adolescence (Compas, Hinden, & Gerhardt, 1995). These have been modified for illustrative purposes and are presented in Fig. 1.3. Some youth display relatively stable adjustment (path 1) or maladjustment (path 5) throughout adolescence. Some start out well but then decline dramatically (path 4); others show marked variability in adjustment, doing better at some times than at others, but eventually ending adolescence as relatively well-adjusted (path 2). Finally, some initially demonstrate poor adjustment but display remarkable improvement over time so that they end adolescence well-adjusted (path 3). These pathways describe the typical sequence for most teens in each group, but some display an alternative path compared to their initial cohort. That is, not every young well-adjusted adolescent demonstrates good adjustment later in adolescence, as path 1 would suggest. Future research may discover more paths occurring in adolescence, but the five pathways presented in Fig. 1.3 illustrate the principles of developmental continuity (paths 1 and 5) and discontinuity (paths 2, 3, and 4).

Figure 1.4 presents the outline of one negative developmental pathway that commonly unfolds in terms of academic functioning. Infants from low-income families are at risk for academic problems because

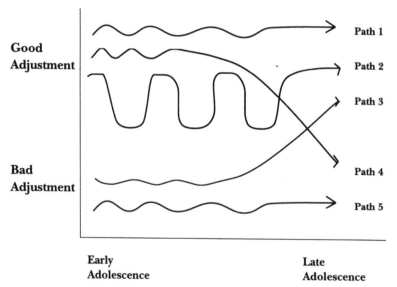

Figure 1.3. Five developmental pathways occurring in adolescence. Modified from Compas, Hinden, and Gerhardt (1995).

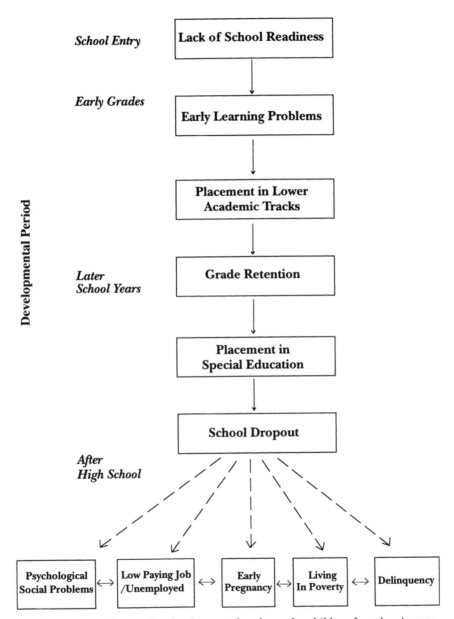

Figure 1.4. Possible negative developmental pathway for children from low-income, high-risk households.

they do not arrive at elementary school prepared or ready to learn (see Chapter 3). Such children demonstrate poor achievement in the early grades and are likely to be placed in lower academic tracks. Learning problems magnify and children fall farther and farther behind; then they are retained in grade, sometimes more than once. Subsequently, they are at higher risk for placement in special education classes, and this event, in turn, increases the risk for dropping out of school. In turn, school dropouts are at greater risk for a host of negative outcomes such as early pregnancy, delinquency, various forms of personal and social maladjustment, having an unskilled job or being unemployed, and living in poverty.

Several interventions that have successfully prevented learning problems essentially have shifted high-risk children from a negative to a positive developmental path. This can be done via early preschool programs that prepare children for school entry, by intensive intervention in the first grade, or by a combination of these approaches. Such interventions are discussed in Chapter 3.

Finally, the pathways in Fig. 1.5 depict three possible consequences of undergoing a stressful life transition. Following the transition: (1) adjustment is enhanced in some way, perhaps because of the way the transition was handled (path 1); (2) there was no change in level of adjustment (path 2); or (3) new problems appear or existing ones intensify suggesting the beginning of a negative trajectory (path 3). Therefore, reasonable goals for a transition intervention are to insure that as many children as possible end up on path 1 and avoid path 3.

Knowing which paths adolescents may take is only part of the story; it is also important to understand the specific developmental processes

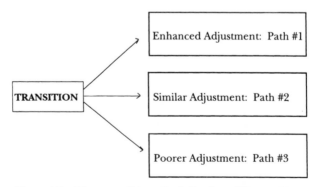

Figure 1.5.   Three possible paths following a life transition.

that explain these paths. It is likely that the five adolescent pathways described by Compas et al. (1995) are associated with different combinations of risk and protective factors, and knowing how these factors operate over time would help preventionists mount more effective intervention programs. Pathways are most helpful when they contain specific information on the sequence of events leading to eventual outcomes and elucidate any critical shifts occurring between positive or negative developmental trajectories.

Systematic Skills Training

A final major theme in prevention has been a shift in the importance of individual factors. Prevention in many different areas began with the assumption that changing knowledge would change behavior. For example, it was believed that if youth had correct information about drugs, sexuality, stress, the importance of finishing school, and so on, this information would motivate them to change their behavior. It is now clear that such prevention programs were based on faulty assumptions. Telling youth how to change their behavior or using fear appeals regarding the dangers that might befall them if they did not act differently has not consistently led to significant behavior change in any area of prevention. This conclusion will be revisited in several chapters of this volume.

Preventionists now recognize that systematic skill training is needed to develop prevention-related behaviors and, furthermore, that mechanisms must be put into place to support and reinforce behavioral change after it occurs. Many successful prevention programs have used social learning principles to teach children and adolescents new skills. Appendix A provides more information on the features of effective skill-training programs.

BRIEF HISTORY OF PREVENTION

Early History

Prevention is not a new idea. Prevention has at least a 100-year-old history in the United States, and young people have always been seen as prime targets for preventive efforts. Although the same terms were not used, early efforts at prevention foreshadowed many of the same principles and concepts as contemporary programs, including a focus on health promotion, early intervention, targeting of high-risk groups, and environmental interventions designed to modify the home, school, and community. For instance, the superintendents of mental asylums during the nineteenth century believed that young children were at high risk for problems and that their upbringing and education should receive special attention (Spaulding & Balch, 1983). During the mid- to late-1800s, organizations such as the National Conference of Charity and Corrections and the Charity Organization Society were formed and began to emphasize early intervention for children and their families (Hetznecker & Forman, 1971). These organizations later evolved into professions we now know as social work and family service.

During the Progressive era in the United States, which occurred roughly from 1890 to the beginning of World War I, many social reformers, volunteers, and charitable organizations were successful in shaping public policy to support programs for children and families. As a result, preventive health programs were developed that involved medical screening and inspections, free medical and dental care for indigent populations, and health education training for teachers and schoolchildren. The Progressive era also launched the first subsidized or free school-based breakfasts and lunches, special classes for handicapped and sick children, counseling for youth and their families, and various vocational programs (Tyack, 1992). Many large cities also developed vacation schools that were eventually transformed into academically oriented summer schools. Originally, however, vacation schools functioned as extended day care and recreational and social development programs during summer periods.

History of Prevention in Mental Health

In 1908, the publication of Clifford Beers' book, *A Mind That Found Itself*, started the mental hygiene movement, which emphasized better care for the mentally ill and the importance of prevention. Beers founded the National Committee of Mental Hygiene in 1909, now known as the National Mental Health Association (NMHA). NMHA is a large volunteer citizen organization that serves a major public health role. NMHA has stimulated the formation of over 500 state and local chapters that have always had three major goals: better treatment of the mentally ill, prevention, and mental health promotion. In 1910, the New York chapter sponsored the first public conference on the prevention of insanity (Long, 1989).

One popular element of the mental hygiene movement was the child guidance clinic, a multidisciplinary agency devoted to serving children and their families. Child clinics spread quickly throughout the United States; from 10 clinics in 1921, the numbers rose to 72 in 1926, to 500 in 1930, and to 617 at the height of the movement in 1935 (Richardson, 1989). Unfortunately, child guidance clinics never achieved their ambitious initial objective which was to emphasize prevention by targeting high-risk groups living in poor neighborhoods and improving children's lives through environmental and social change. Instead, most clinics primarily offered individual long-term treatment to children from middle- and upper-class families (Hetznecker & Forman, 1971; Horn, 1989).

Nonetheless, a few early child guidance programs were impressive. One demonstration project in New York offered fellowships to social work students wishing to learn preventive concepts through fieldwork experiences. Eventually, a coordinated, community-based intervention program was developed that involved 18 schools, 4 churches, 5 hospitals, and 23 different social agencies (Richardson, 1989).

School Programs

Several preventively oriented school programs also appeared. In the 1920s, specially trained visiting teachers (the historical forerunners of school social workers) entered classrooms to educate regular teachers on preventive concepts. Visiting teachers demonstrated ways to develop positive personal and social qualities in students (what we would now call social skills), acted as ombudspersons for families to help them obtain needed resources and services, and were active in modifying the school environment to promote social and academic growth (Horn, 1989). Preventive curricula taught by regular classroom teachers and designed to enhance self-esteem and improve social functioning began to appear during the early 1940s; special intervention programs were also developed for high-risk schoolchildren (Long, 1989).

The 1950s and 1960s

The period between 1950 and 1970 represents a time of some interest but relatively little activity in prevention. In the 1960s, community mental health centers (CMHCs) became part of a national plan in the United States to offer community-based mental health services throughout the country. Each community center was to have a multidisciplinary staff and to deal comprehensively with the mental health needs of local populations. Many professionals saw tremendous potential in CMHCs and believed that services for children should receive priority. Just like the child guidance clinics before them, CMHCs spread rapidly from approximately 130 centers in 1966 to over 700 centers by 1979. However, most CMHCs emphasized treatment and did not do much prevention.

To receive federal funding, CMHCs had to offer five essential mental health services, but prevention was not one of them. Many centers never became staffed with personnel who had expertise with children, in prevention, or in community-based intervention. As a result, traditional forms of treatment constituted the bulk of services offered by most centers. Few centers attempted prevention and services for children were frequently shortchanged (Berlin, 1990). Prevention also suffered at the federal level. Between 1967 to 1979, there was only one professional in the National Institute of Mental Health responsible for activities related to primary prevention and there was no designated prevention budget (Goldston, 1986).

Current History of Prevention

During the past 25 years, the pendulum has swung back toward heightened activity in prevention. Several factors have coalesced to promote prevention: (1) growing recognition that it is difficult to treat many problems once they are established; (2) limitations in the delivery of services that leave many in need without any help; and (3) optimism that prevention may be a cost-effective approach in solving social problems. Perhaps the greatest influence, however, has been the findings from several well-done studies that prevention is both doable and effective. Scores of programs have reported success in reducing child and adolescent problems and in promoting adjustment, and this exciting literature is examined throughout this volume.

A History Lesson

There is one important lesson that history teaches about prevention: The failure to secure ongoing administrative and financial support for programs threatens their long-term viability. There are several historical examples of prevention programs born as pilot or demonstration projects that were discontinued when their initial sources of support ended despite the success of the intervention (Horn, 1989; Richardson, 1989). The same thing may occur with many of today's programs unless they are well-integrated and incorporated into existing health and social care systems. We will return to this point in the last chapter.

Current Research and Practice on Prevention

Research

Depictions of the adoption or spread of social and technological innovations over time frequently result in S-shaped growth curves (Hamblin, Jacobsen, & Miller, 1973). That is, new innovations spread slowly at first, then rapidly and exponentially, and finally growth levels off after they have been tested or used in many settings. An S-shaped growth curve can also be seen in the number of outcome studies on prevention that have been published. Figure 1.6 covers the period from 1956 through the end of 1995. The data are presented in 5-year time blocks and reflect how only a few publications appeared between 1956 and 1965, followed by a rapid increase in publications between 1975 and 1995.[3] There have been at least 1200 published outcome studies of preventive interventions. Yet, prevention is a very young science; 90.4% of all studies appeared after 1975, and 30.5% ($n = 367$) appeared after 1990.

Practice

As is true with many other social programs or innovations, the practice of prevention goes far beyond its research base. That is, many more programs are conducted than are systematically evaluated in any fashion. This is clear from surveys of private and public school curricula that indicate that some instruction in prevention is offered in almost all elementary, junior high, and high schools and many schools offer multiple programs (Collins et al., 1995). The topics covered and the percentage of schools including each topic is as follows: alcohol and other drugs (90%), tobacco use (86%), HIV prevention (86%), diet and nutrition (84%), sexually transmitted disease prevention (84%), human sexuality (80%), emotional and mental health (74%), pregnancy prevention (69%), injury prevention and personal safety (66%), conflict resolution or violence prevention (58%), and suicide prevention (58%). Further-

[3]The studies in Fig. 1.6 were drawn from an extensive, although not exhaustive, search of English-language journal articles and books in the areas covered in this book such as mental health, drug programs, and physical health. The count in Fig. 1.6 is conservative. Only controlled outcome studies were counted; case reports, programs lacking within-subject or between-subject experimental controls, and qualitative commentaries were not included. Furthermore, there are probably an equal number of unpublished reports on prevention. Slavin, Karweit, and Wasik (1994) examined over 500 unpublished reports of programs designed to prevent academic problems.

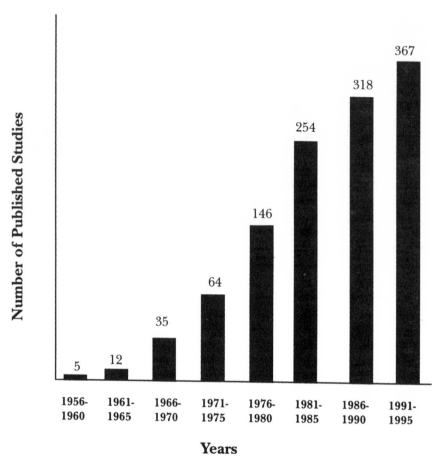

Figure 1.6. Number of published outcome studies on prevention from 1956 through the end of 1995.

more, over 90% of all school districts receive federal funding to help children at risk for academic problems (Slavin, Karweit, & Madden, 1989). In effect, each year millions of schoolchildren are exposed to preventive programs of one form of another and most are exposed to more than one. The type and intensity of prevention programming vary greatly across schools and topics and may range from a single class lesson to a comprehensive multigrade curriculum.

Many community-based programs also exist. Parents participate in up to 3000 community-based drug prevention programs (Klitzner,

Gruenwald, & Bamberger, 1990); at least 600 agencies offer sex abuse prevention (Kohl, 1993); there are an untold number of additional interventions offered by social agencies and health organizations; and about two thirds of all businesses with over 50 employees sponsor preventively oriented health and wellness programs (Simmons, 1993).

Because so many programs exist, it is important to identify which ones are effective. This is not a research text on prevention, although it is thoroughly grounded on empirical findings. I do not concentrate on the methodological complexities involved in prevention research, which are discussed elsewhere (Heller, Price, & Sher, 1980; Institute of Medicine, 1994; Jason, Thompson & Rose, 1986). However, in an effort to describe successful prevention programs, I have selected those interventions that have the strongest empirical support. The programs cited throughout this volume represent those that have been carefully conceptualized, executed, and evaluated. These interventions thus serve as exemplars in their respective fields. No single study is perfect, of course, but the science of prevention is rapidly evolving, and some areas are in their fourth or fifth generation of research as investigators continue to refine and improve prior work.

In addition, I focus on interventions that have changed behavior, since behavior change in the sine qua non of effective prevention. As the previous discussion on skill training has indicated, it is insufficient to know if participants have more knowledge about prevention as a result of intervention. What we really wish to know is whether their behavior and adjustment status change.

We also need to understand the extent of change that is produced by prevention. Does prevention have a practical effect on children's lives? Statistically significant research findings can occur, but outcomes may have little meaningful social or practical significance. This is an important issue, so that whenever possible the magnitude of changes emanating from prevention and their practical implications are highlighted. Fortunately, there have been many programs that have produced substantial positive changes in children's and adolescents' lives.

In summary, this volume presents a panoramic snapshot of prevention with an emphasis on the very best programs. The main theme of this volume is that prevention works in the sense that many programs produce significant and meaningful reductions in future problems, improvements in adaptive functioning, or both, and that these gains are often maintained over time. Not every intervention is effective, however, so there is a need to identify the factors and circumstances associated with program success. As a result, in addition to giving the reader an appreciation for the procedures and outcomes of programs conducted in different areas, whenever possible I offer insights into what seems to make interventions effective.

Successful prevention programs have been conducted throughout the world. Unless otherwise indicated, information presented in this volume refers to the United States, but data collected in the following countries are also represented: Australia, Canada, China, Colombia, Finland, France, Germany, Great Britain, India, Ireland, Israel, Japan, Netherlands, Norway, Singapore, South Korea, Spain, Sweden, Taiwan, and Turkey.

PLAN OF THE BOOK

There are ten chapters in this book. This first chapter has defined primary and secondary (indicated) prevention and described several approaches and themes central to prevention. The following chapters summarize the procedures and results of exemplary programs in different areas. Chapter 2 describes efforts to prevent behavioral and social problems; Chapter 3 discusses the prevention of learning problems; and Chapter 4 focuses on preventing the use of cigarettes, alcohol, and other drugs. Chapter 5 discusses programs to improve physical health, with sections devoted to programs for mothers with young children, elementary school-aged populations, and interventions devoted to AIDS and sex education and the prevention of pregnancy. The prevention of injuries and child maltreatment (physical and sexual abuse) is covered in Chapters 6 and 7, respectively. Chapter 8 takes up the important matter of cost-effectiveness and discusses issues related to determining the relative costs and benefits of different interventions. In Chapter 9, the role and preventive impact of representative policy initiatives are discussed. Finally, Chapter 10 summarizes the current status of prevention for children and adolescents and discusses the future. Appendix A summarizes the principles of effective skill-training programs, and Appendix B contains additional sources of information on prevention such as books, journals, and national clearinghouses that distribute relevant information.

SUMMARY

Prevention is a multidisciplinary science that draws from at least 15 major fields of study and several subspecialties within these fields. Prevention is a very young science and most research has been con-

ducted within the past 20 years. In general, preventionists seek to understand the developmental processes occurring in the pathways that lead
to positive and negative outcomes and then intervene to influence these
outcomes. Primary prevention may be defined as a set of approaches
including health promotion that are designed to prevent future problems in currently normal populations by modifying individuals, their
environments, or both. Indicated (secondary) prevention uses a corresponding set of approaches to prevent more serious problems from
developing in those who are demonstrating early difficulties. There are
three major ways that populations are selected for intervention (universal, high-risk, and transition approaches) and five possible levels of
intervention (individual, family, peer, school, and community). These
approaches can be combined in various ways. Five important themes
guide preventive interventions: multiple causality, the importance of
risk and protection (positive) factors, health promotion, developmental
pathways, and systematic skill training.

2

Prevention of Behavioral and Social Problems

INTRODUCTION

Many children and adolescents are affected by mental health problems of one kind or another. Between 17 to 22% of youth up to age 18 develop a clinical disorder, that is, a behavioral or emotional problem that significantly impairs their personal or social adjustment and warrants treatment (Kazdin, 1990), and between 12 to 53% who have one disorder also have at least one other co-occurring disorder (Nottelmann & Jensen, 1995). In addition to these clinical conditions, another 15 to 25% of young people could profit from intervention because they experience interpersonal deficits, sadness, or lack of self-control or self-confidence that impedes their personal and social growth.

Unfortunately, the mental health needs of most children are unmet. For a variety of reasons, most clinically distressed youth (70–90%) never receive any formal treatment, and when treatment is provided it may be too brief to be of much help. For instance, a majority of schoolchildren who have the most serious emotional problems receive less than five sessions of therapy a year (Knitzer, Steinberg, & Fleisch, 1990), and mental health programs are rarely developed for mildly impaired youth.

Furthermore, young people are increasingly becoming either victims or perpetrators of crime and violence. In addition to the over 1 million children who are the documented victims of child abuse (see Chapter 7), another 3.3 million children witness or are otherwise exposed to other forms of domestic violence (American Psychological Association, 1996).

Approximately 3 million crimes occur at or near schools each year. This translates into 16,000 crimes a day, or one crime every 6 seconds! An estimated 4% of high school students report carrying guns to school, 15% carry knives, and 3% carry clubs; half of all 10th graders report they could obtain a handgun if they wanted one (Coben, Weiss, Mulvey, & Dearwater, 1994).

One out of every 16 adolescents are victims of violent crime annually, and homicide has become the leading cause of death among African Americans and Latinos under 25 (Soriano, Soriano, & Jimenez, 1994). Over a 10-year period from 1982 through 1991, juvenile arrest rates rose 24% for forcible rape, 72% for aggravated assault, and 93% for murder (Bennett, 1994). Psychological problems and high rates of crime and violence create a troubling mix of conditions for today's youth that can jeopardize their growth and development.

In addition to the many problems and stresses affecting children and adolescents, positive mental health should not be ignored. Many youth never develop a strong sense of psychological well-being, high self-esteem, or the coping and social skills that are within their potential. In summary, much can be done to reduce maladjustment and promote mental health in young people.

PRIMARY PREVENTION PROGRAMS

Durlak and Wells (1997a) evaluated 177 controlled outcome studies of primary prevention mental health programs designed to prevent behavioral and social problems in children and adolescents. There were several different categories of programs attempting different goals, and analyses indicated that most types of programs obtained significant positive outcomes. Mean effect sizes averaged across all types of outcome measures for the successful programs ranged from 0.24 to 0.93.[1] Furthermore, most programs had the dual benefit of significantly reducing problems and significantly increasing competencies. Fig. 2.1 summarizes the mean effects obtained at postprogram and at follow-up across all programs for different types of outcomes.

---

[1]An effect size is a standardized statistic that reflects the superiority of the intervention group over the control group; higher numbers indicate better outcomes. The majority of mean effects (68%) obtained from psychological, medical, and educational interventions fall somewhere between 0.19 and 0.75 (Lipsey & Wilson, 1993).

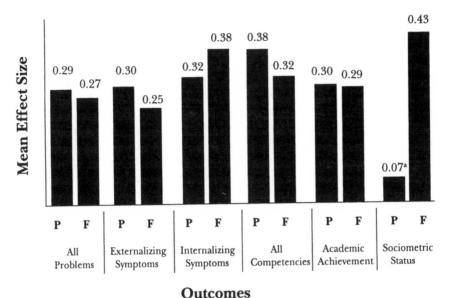

Outcomes

Figure 2.1. Post (P) and follow-up (F) mean effect sizes for primary prevention mental health programs across different outcome domains. Data are from Durlak and Wells (1997a). [a] = Only mean effect size not significantly different from zero.

The outcome category, All Competencies, refers to measures assessing changes in such areas as academic functioning, self-esteem or self-confidence, and various social skills such as communication and assertiveness. The category, All Problems, contains different types of externalizing or internalizing problems.[2] Outcomes for some major subcategories of competencies and problems are also presented in Fig. 2.1. The postprogram mean effect sizes for sociometric status is the only finding that failed to reach statistical significance.

The range of effects achieved in primary prevention programs is impressive. Participants in primary prevention programs are, by definition, already functioning in the normal range. Therefore, reductions in

---

[2]Externalizing problems, also called disruptive, acting-out, or undercontrolled problems, reflect lack of appropriate self-control and include aggression, stealing, lying, noncompliance, and delinquent acts. Internalizing problems are characterized by high degrees of subjective distress and overcontrolled behavior and include anxiety, depression, social inhibition or isolation, and somatic complaints.

both internalizing and externalizing symptomatology refer to subclinical level difficulties. Although program participants do not have much room to change in this regard, they nevertheless demonstrate significant reductions in various problems or symptoms. On the positive side, both academic functioning and social competencies are important predictors of future adjustment, and interventions have achieved positive effects in these dimensions as well. The overall impression is that mental health programs seem able to both reduce risk (lessen problems) and increase protection (increase competencies) in target populations. Several authors have offered useful recommendations to improve current programs (Sandler, 1997). Meanwhile, current outcome data support the value of primary prevention mental health programs.

The following sections describe different programs using the conceptual scheme presented in Chapter 1. In other words, person-centered and environment-centered programs, examples of mental health promotion, and programs conducted at different transition times are described to give the reader a sense of intervention accomplishments and the variety of approaches undertaken to achieve different goals.

Person-Centered Programs

A research team at Johns Hopkins (Dolan et al., 1993; Kellam, Rebok, Ialongo, & Mayer, 1994) developed a successful intervention to prevent aggressive behavior among multiethnic, inner-city children attending Baltimore public schools. This group demonstrated the preventive value of the Good Behavior Game (GBG), which uses group contingencies to modify children's classroom behavior. The procedure is generally deployed as follows. The teacher divides the class into teams, being careful to distribute children who have difficulty controlling their behavior on to different teams, and then defines for the class what types of behaviors will not be tolerated (such as verbal and physical disruption, noncompliance, and so on). When GBG was played, any time a child violated one of the class rules, that child's team received a tally or checkmark that was posted for all to see. Children won the game when their team did not exceed a specified number of tallies. All children on winning teams received a small reward for winning the game and all teams could win.

The advantage of GBG is its flexibility. The teacher can determine when the game is played, for how long, what the criterion is for winning, and what rewards are possible. Over time, the behavioral criteria and duration of the game are usually modified to match the children's behavioral improvement. GBG is believed to work because the procedure provides an effective group contingency for enhancing children's self-control and prompts children to help others control their behavior.

In the Baltimore study, GBG had a significant positive effect on levels of aggressive behavior by the end of first grade (Dolan et al., 1993). Four-year follow-up data (Kellam et al., 1994) indicated that the intervention was successful in reducing rates of aggressive behavior for males who initially had the highest rates of aggressive behavior in first grade. In other words, the program had long-term positive effects on those at highest risk. GBG did not affect girls' aggressive behavior, but their initial level of aggression was generally low to begin with; that is, there was not much room for girls to change on this dimension.

Mental Health Promotion

Several person-centered programs have chosen various mental health promotion strategies. For example, some have taught rational emotive therapy (RET) mental health principles to schoolchildren. RET emphasizes the importance of controlling or correcting irrational cognitions that can produce negative feelings and behavior. RET programs have been helpful for both middle school (Digiuseppe & Kassinove, 1976) and high school students (Ross, 1978) in reducing anxiety, irrational thinking, and neuroticism.

Affective education interventions have also been used successfully in several studies. Affective education generally refers to a wide range of interventions that teach children how to become more aware of their own and others' feelings and how to understand the possible intentions that guide behavior. Some of the earliest successful primary prevention programs involved affective education (Ojemann, Levitt, Lyle, & Whiteside, 1955). Among more current programs, DeCharms (1972) evaluated the impact of one form of affective education, called personal causation training, on African-American elementary students. The training was designed to help children understand their strengths and weaknesses and set realistic personal goals. Teachers conducted the intervention in their classrooms over a 2-year period, and the program produced positive changes in children's personal responsibility and goal-setting behavior. There were also concomitant positive changes in children's school absences and tardiness and improvement in boys' language and arithmetic skills.

Finally, interpersonal problem-solving training is another widely used promotion strategy. Most programs have been influenced by

Spivack and Shure's (1974) work suggesting that improving problem-solving skills improves children's adjustment and reduces behavioral problems. Problem-solving programs take several different forms but generally focus on training children on one or more the following dimensions: (1) how to recognize the existence of interpersonal problems; (2) how to develop multiple possible solutions to these problems; and (3) and how to think through the consequences of different strategies before acting. Outcomes for interventions other than those conducted by the Spivack and Shure research group have been mixed, although problem-solving training has been a part of several successful multi-component programs. Future research needs to clarify the specific impact of problem-solving training.

Transition Programs

Four categories of transition programs have achieved positive outcomes: programs for first-time mothers, for children entering or changing schools, for children of divorce, and for those undergoing stressful medical and dental treatments. Examples in each of these areas are presented below.

First-Time Parents

One successful program was the Pittsburgh First-Born Project (Broussard, 1982) which combined home visits and clinic group meetings. Groups met biweekly to provide education and support for first-time mothers; meetings began when the infants were 2–4 months old and lasted until the children were 3½ years olds. Home visits conducted by child care specialists were interspersed among these group meetings. The intervention led to a significant improvement in children's overall psychosocial functioning.

A Dutch home visiting program (van den Boom, 1995) taught new mothers how to monitor their infant's signals and respond appropriately and contingently to infant behavior. The intermediate goal was to promote secure infant attachment, which, it was hoped, would lay the groundwork for a good parent–child relationship that would foster child development. Mothers giving birth to temperamentally irritable infants, who were considered to be at high risk for developing less secure attachments, were visited in their homes over a 3-month period. Home observations confirmed that compared to controls, program mothers were significantly more responsive, stimulating, soothing, and attentive to their infants. More than twice as many program than control infants were securely attached at 18 months of age (72 vs. 26%, respectively). A 33-month follow-up found that intervention mothers continued to be significantly more responsive and helpful to their toddlers, who demonstrated significantly more appropriate and fewer problem behaviors during peer interactions.

School Entry and Change

Probably the most frequent transition experienced by children is a school transition. It is estimated that approximately 6 million children between the ages of 5 and 13 change schools each year (Jason et al., 1992). Most children change schools several times during their life; for instance, only 20% or so remain in the same school during all of their elementary school years. Although not all children are affected negatively by school transitions, many children will experience some problems and some never seem to make a good adjustment.

A series of studies has confirmed the value of the School Transition Project (STP), developed by Jason and his colleagues at DePaul University, Chicago (Jason et al., 1992). STP is based on an ecological model that suggests that the adjustment process of transfer students depends on both individual and environmental factors and their interaction over time. STP emphasizes such individual factors as the child's prior academic and emotional adjustment and their coping skills, and environmental factors such as the presence of stressful life events and social support provided by peers, school staff, and parents.

One important component of STP is a special orientation program held for all new students conducted by a sixth grade peer leader at the new school. This orientation covers aspects of the new school's environment and policies and provides new students with a chance to ask questions. Peer buddies are assigned to provide continuing informational and emotional support to new students and to help them enter a new peer group. Some research on school transitions suggests that school staff may underestimate both the degree and nature of stresses experienced by new students (Elias, Gara, & Umbriaco, 1985). Therefore, STP also wisely contains an informational component for school staff to alert them to typical problems encountered by transfer students.

Other core features of STP include school- and home-based tutoring program conducted by paid paraprofessional staff or by parents, respectively. The paraprofessionals also work as child advocates within the school system and as liaisons to help parents become more involved in their child's school life. An important accomplishment in STP has been securing the participation of 95% of target parents for the home tutoring program. Few other school-based programs have achieved this level of success in involving parents.

STP has worked with several groups of ethnically and culturally diverse urban school children and has identified high-risk groups of transfer students based on a combination of three factors: lower socio-economic status, the presence of many recent stressful life events, and lower previous achievement scores. One program evaluation reflected two important findings: (1) STP students improved significantly more than controls on measures of academic achievement; and (2) 50% more STP students than control students were no longer considered to be at high-risk following program participation. Other evaluations indicate that teachers report decreased social withdrawal and inattentiveness among transfer students, and the academic gains manifested by STP children continue to be maintained at 1-year follow-up.

Combining measures of academic achievement and social status based on peer ratings, it was possible to categorize transfer students who had good, average, or poor coping skills (Jason, Johnson, Danner, Taylor, & Kurasaki, 1993). Focusing on the poor coping group and comparing STP children to matched controls, school tutoring was associated with 42% more STP students moving out of the poor coping category after intervention; a school tutoring plus home tutoring condition was even more successful; 90% more program students moved out of the poor coping category. Such data illustrate the ability of STP to influence the adjustment status of high risk groups.

Children of Divorce

Divorce is affecting more and more children. It is estimated that by age 16, 33% of white children and 75% of African-American children will experience at least one parental divorce, and martial conflict and the divorce process can negatively affect children in many different ways (Emery & Forehand, 1994).

A series of studies have indicated the value of the Children of Divorce Intervention Program (CODIP) (Pedro-Carroll & Cowen, 1985). CODIP is a relatively brief (10–16 sessions) school-based group intervention designed to provide children of divorce with peer support, to educate them about divorce and clarify their misconceptions (e.g., children are to blame for the divorce), to facilitate expression of feelings, and finally to teach relevant coping skills. A series of games and exercises is designed to achieve these purposes, and procedures vary depending on the child's age and developmental status. Children from grades 2 through 6 have displayed significant improvements in competent classroom behaviors and corresponding reductions in internalizing and externalizing problems. Children also report less anxiety and more positive divorce-related attitudes and perceptions. Parents report significantly fewer behavioral problems at home.

A second program is the Divorce Adjustment Project (DAP) (Stolberg & Mahler, 1994). DAP includes parental involvement in its intervention based on the belief that parental reactions to the child's behavior and emotions mediate children's adjustment to divorce. Program evaluations have evaluated separate interventions emphasizing social support alone, social support plus skill building, and both of these combined with parent involvement. DAP uses parent workbooks linked to the progress of school-based group sessions to encourage parents to extend the intervention into the home environment. Parents are asked to initiate conversations about divorce-related topics and to provide support and understanding to their child. Overall, DAP has led to significant improvements in children's school and home functioning. At follow-up, the greatest gains occurred in the intervention that combines support, skill building, and parent involvement.

Dental and Medical Treatment

Another life event that can have negative effects on large numbers of children is dental or medical treatment, particularly treatment that involves hospitalization or surgery. Approximately 5% of all children enter hospitals each year, and it has been estimated that anywhere from 10 to 36% of children display relatively severe problems, and up to 90% of young children will demonstrate increased anxiety and behavioral distress in response to various medical or dental procedures (Harbeck-Weber & McKee, 1995; Yap, 1988). Transition programs for medical and dental patients have been effective in reducing anxiety and behavioral problems (mean effect size = 0.46) (Durlak & Wells, 1997a).

Many programs have successfully used modeling, desensitization, and coping skills training. Live or filmed models illustrate upcoming procedures and demonstrate that children can cope successfully with such treatment without undue negative consequences. In some studies, children have been taught deep muscle relaxation or have been trained in various imagery and self-control strategies.

Current research findings have implications for the redesign of many existing hospital preparation programs that are conducted on the belief that information presented in very brief sessions or through take-home materials will prevent future anxiety and behavioral distress. Research data indicate that such informational techniques produce, at best, very modest effects, and that more skill-oriented interventions such as those involving modeling or coping skills training are much more helpful for children. For example, Melamed and Siegel (1975) compared the effects of one hospital's usual informational preparation procedures with a filmed modeling condition showing a child patient dealing effectively with the same upcoming treatments. According to parent reports, children receiving the usual hospital preparation demonstrated an *increase* in behavior problems when they returned home following hospitalization for minor surgery. Children seeing the modeling film displayed no such increase over time, suggesting that the modeling condition had prevented the occurrence of subsequent problems. Another research group (Peterson, Schultheis, Ridley-Johnson, Miller, & Tracy, 1984) compared the effects of filmed modeling with another hospital's informational preparation procedures and found that children who viewed the films demonstrated significantly less anxiety and distress than no-treatment controls.

Environment-Centered Programs

Environment-centered mental health programs assume many forms but generally have sought to modify the psychosocial characteristics of either the school or home environment (and sometimes both) by changing the ways that teachers and parents interact with children. The basic idea behind these interventions is that changing the behavior of significant others will lead to positive changes in child behavior. Children may receive some direct services in these programs, but a primary thrust is to modify the child's behavior indirectly by changing adult behavior.

School-Based Programs

The School Transitions Environment Project (STEP) simultaneously attempts to reduce stress levels and increase interpersonal support for high-risk students transferring to junior high or high school (Felner et al., 1993).[3] This is accomplished in two major ways. First, the school's academic curriculum is refashioned by assigning incoming students to homerooms consisting of between 20 to 30 students and

[3]STEP illustrates how the different categorical approaches to primary prevention discussed in Chapter 1 can overlap. STEP can be placed into any of three different categories noted in Fig. 1.1: a high-risk approach, an environmental-level intervention, or a transitions approach.

having the students in these homerooms remain together for at least four of their core academic classes during the school day. This allows new students to develop more stable friendships among peers who are facing similar academic and social demands. Second, the supportive school environment is enhanced by expanding the role of the homeroom teachers who now assume advisory and counseling functions for their students. Teachers offer personal guidance and advice as needed and become part of a school team to monitor students' academic and personal adjustment. Teachers may intervene to obtain additional school services or increase parents' involvement in school life. STEP teachers appear to like their expanded roles and the opportunity to interact with other teachers in a team approach, suggesting that STEP may be well-received and replicable in other school settings.

Evaluations indicate that STEP prevents deterioration in grades, attendance, and levels of self-concept. Although at-risk control students entering new schools tend to show such problems, STEP students do not. STEP has significantly improved students' classroom behavior and adjustment, as reflected by teacher ratings, and reduced students' self-reported levels of general stress, depression, anxiety, and delinquent behavior (Felner et al., 1993). Data also suggest that the school environment has been changed positively for STEP students. Compared to controls, STEP students report that their school is more stable, well-organized, and supportive. Finally, STEP has had substantial, practical, long-term effects. A 4-year follow-up indicated that by the 12th grade, school dropout rates were 55.58% lower for STEP than for control students. Analyses of absenteeism and levels of academic achievement also confirmed that STEP students were doing significantly better during high school than their control counterparts. These findings are particularly noteworthy, since the original study sample consisted of many minority students from low-socioeconomic households who were considered at high risk for later school problems.

Peer Bullying

A series of investigations (summarized in Olweus, 1994) has focused on one form of aggressive peer behavior called bullying. Bullying occurs when children are physically or verbally assaulted and threatened by peers. Data indicate that approximately one out of every seven Norwegian school-age children are affected; 9% are the victims of bullying, 7% admit to bullying others, and approximately 2% are both

the initiators and recipients of bullying tactics.[4] Bullying is more common among boys than girls, and is associated with impulsivity, positive
views toward violence, and a likelihood to display other aggressive
behaviors. Therefore, bullying is one behavioral risk factor associated
with later more serious aggressive and antisocial behavior.

The approach developed by Olweus to prevent bullying is a multicomponent intervention targeting the individual, the family, the teacher,
and the entire school. Basically, intervention begins with the school
adopting a policy to combat bullying and then instituting several initiatives to implement this policy. The two main principles underlying
intervention are that adults at school and in the home must communicate warmth and acceptance of children and at the same time provide
clear and prompt sanctions for any aggressive behavior. Individuals
who bully receive personal counseling and parent training is also offered if needed. The other components attempt to change social norms
and rewards regarding interpersonal behavior. Parents and teachers are
educated regarding the incidence and impact of bullying through book-
lets, workshops, and conferences. School staff develop procedures to
supervise and monitor child behavior during school and also work with
parents to monitor children's behavior between school and home.
Teachers are encouraged to establish class rules sanctioning bullying
and praising positive peer behaviors, and class meetings are regularly
convened to deal with specific behavioral incidents.

Antibullying programs have been developed in many Scandinavian
school districts and results have been encouraging. Rates of bullying
have fallen by as much as 50%, and other forms of antisocial or aggressive behavior such as vandalism, fighting, stealing, and truancy have
also been reduced. The intervention is also successful in changing the
school's social atmosphere. Students report improved attitudes toward
and satisfaction with school and their social relationships.

Olweus (1994) reported that better outcomes are obtained the longer
a program is in operation. Such findings have important implications.
The impact of some preventive interventions might not be completely
obvious until the program has been in place for some time. Thus, there is
the danger of dismissing a preventive program prematurely because it
does not lead to immediate dramatic results. Prevention must be given

[4]Peer bullying is a problem in many societies. In the United States, between 12 to 15% of
youth report being the victim of peer bullying (Finkelhor & Dziuba-Leatherman, 1994;
Nolin, Davies, & Chandler, 1996). Japanese statistics indicated 56,000 documented cases
of peer bullying during 1995, and the pressure and stress resulting from bullying was
implicated in at least 10 childhood suicides (Lev, 1996).

sufficient time to exert its effects, particularly if the intervention attempts to modify multiple aspects of the environment that are difficult to change quickly.

The Social Development Program (SDP) is another environment-centered program that combines school- and home-based components. (Hawkins et al., 1991). SDP seeks to reduce later rates of aggression, delinquency, and drug use by developing prosocial attachments in young children. Teachers and parents are taught how to reward children for prosocial behavior. SDP is an intensive multicomponent program beginning when children enter first grade. Parents participate in SDP by attending training sessions to learn behaviorally oriented methods emphasizing consistency of discipline and reinforcement for positive behaviors. Concurrently, teachers are implementing several new interventions in school. Teachers learn proactive classroom management techniques that help them manage and direct children's classroom behavior more efficiently. Teachers also learn to use mastery-oriented teaching practices that emphasize reinforcement for step-by-step academic progress. Cooperative learning principles are also implemented to enhance the achievement of all students (see Chapter 4 for a discussion of these educational techniques). Finally, teachers also administer a social skills training program in the classroom over the course of the year.

SDP has yielded several positive findings. At the end of a 2-year intervention, there was a significant reduction in aggression among boys and self-destructive behaviors among girls (Hawkins et al., 1991). The percentage of boys subsequently demonstrating clinical levels of aggressive behavior was reduced by 34%. There has also been a 6-year-long replication of the SDP program that obtained significant gains for boys, girls, or both sexes on a variety of outcomes, including attachment to school, rates of classroom participation, school achievement, use of alcohol, marijuana, and tobacco, and delinquent behaviors (O'Donnell, Hawkins, Catalano, Abbott, & Day, 1995).

School Vandalism

Another research group has focused on preventing school vandalism (Mayer & Butterworth, 1979; Mayer, Butterworth, Nafpaktitis, & Sulzer-Azaroff, 1983). Over $500 million dollars each year are spent repairing vandalized school property (National Institute of Education, 1978). The belief was that vandalism could be reduced by making the school environment more positive and reinforcing to students and by increasing students' attachment to their school. In general, this meant deemphasizing punitive techniques in response to student misbehavior and replacing these reactions with systematic positive teaching and management practices. It also meant involving school staff and students in group projects. The methods for two school vandalism studies were similar.

The general idea of the intervention was to first train a core group of motivated staff (e.g., the school principal, school psychologist or counselor, and a few teachers) and then use these personnel as consultants within their own schools to extend the intervention to others. Members of the core group were taught basic reinforcement principles and how to serve as consultants to other school staff. Both classroom and school-wide interventions were stressed. For instance, teachers learned how to match learning materials with student ability levels more effectively, to reinforce student effort and productivity in step-by-step fashion, and to share ideas and problem solve with other teachers. On a school-wide basis, programs were begun in the lunchroom and playground that emphasized positive reinforcement techniques. School clubs were involved in keeping the school campus clean, and they were asked to brainstorm how the school should use any money saved from reduced vandalism costs. This served as a potentially strong incentive for students to work toward preventing vandalism. Neighborhood walks were conducted to inform local residents of the school's effort to reduce vandalism and to enlist their cooperation.

The interventions were successful in modifying teachers' and students' classroom behaviors and in reducing vandalism. In the first study (Mayer & Butterworth, 1979), data were collected in 20 experimental schools and 18 no-treatment control schools. Students' disruptive and nontask classroom behavior decreased and their attending behavior increased over time only in experimental schools. Most important, while the average costs from vandalism increased 320% across control schools, it decreased 57% in experimental schools.

In the second study (Mayer et al., 1983), the behavior of randomly selected teachers at each school who were not initially trained by the research staff was evaluated to see how well the initial intervention had spread to other staff. Teachers' rates of praise increased significantly and the off-task classroom behavior of their students decreased significantly following treatment. Vandalism costs were also reduced by an average of 78.5% in project schools over time. Supplemental data indicated that school staff reported fewer discipline problems, greater cooperation, and better relationships among students and staff. These latter more impressionistic findings suggest that the overall school climate was positively affected by the intervention.

Creating New Settings

Another multifaceted, environmentally oriented program that was designed to improve family functioning as a way to prevent future behavioral problems has involved the creation of a new community agency, the Houston Parent–Child Development Center (HPCDC) (Johnson, 1988). HPCDC is notable in several respects: (1) its focus on a low-income Mexican-American population; (2) its intensive character requiring over 550 hours of participants' involvement; and (3) its targeting of the total family, including fathers who are frequently overlooked in family-oriented programs.

HPCDC offers services during the first 3 years of a child's life. During the first year, indigenous bilingual staff make home visits to inform mothers about child development and ways to stimulate their child's cognitive and social growth. Family workshops are also scheduled on weekends to include fathers and focus on decision making and communication within the family. After their first birthday, children enter a 2-year nursery school program at HPCDC for four mornings a week. Several additional family-oriented services are offered concurrent with the nursery school experience. These include English-language classes for parents, community health care programs, parent training sessions, and various homemaking services. HPCDC also offers additional programs that are requested by families such as driver's education, sex education, and family planning. The general intent is to promote multiple aspects of family functioning that will, in turn, foster children's growth and development.

HPCDC outcomes have been impressive. Parents provide a more stimulating educational environment to their children, they praise more and criticize less, and they are less rigidly controlling of their child's behavior. Follow-up evaluations conducted when the children were preschoolers indicate they were less destructive, attention seeking, and overactive; in elementary school (grades 2 to 5), program children had significantly fewer acting-out behaviors.

Parent Training

Programs that relied exclusively on parent training were the only category found by Durlak and Wells (1997a) that did not produce significant overall positive effects (mean effect size, 0.16). These parent programs sought to improve parents' childrearing techniques by using

Rogerian, Adlerian, or behavioral principles and were typically conducted in a group context over a short time period.

It is unknown why parent training by itself has not been effective.
Like problem solving, parent training has been used as one component
in successful multicomponent programs. Interventions for parents
might need to be longer and more intensive to achieve their goals. Self-
selection bias may also be a contributing factor. It has been difficult to
recruit parents for parent training. One program was offered to 1500
parents whose children attended three different elementary schools, but
only 68 parents eventually participated (Frazier & Matthes, 1975). Some
parent programs may be "preaching to the converted" in the sense that
those who eventually participate might be those who least need the
intervention. This has happened in some parent-oriented drug prevention programs (Cohen & Linton, 1995). If the parents who participate in
primary prevention programs are already doing an effective job, there is
little room for them to change, and program outcomes are likely to be
discouraging. Because parents play such a central role in children's
lives, preventionists must devise effective ways of involving more parents who can benefit from intervention. For example, offering home-
based services has been effective in some cases (e.g., Johnson, 1988; van
den Boom, 1995) and offering parent programs at the workplace has
been effective in others (e.g., Colan, Mague, Cohen, & Schneider, 1994;
Felner et al., 1994).

INDICATED (SECONDARY) PREVENTION

General Overview

In an indicated prevention approach, the idea is to intervene with
populations that are showing early signs of dysfunction to prevent the
occurrence of later clinical disorders or more serious problems. Such
approaches rest upon three important assumptions: (1) youth with
subclinical-level difficulties can be identified; (2) those with early problems are at risk for later more serious difficulties; and (3) early intervention will improve adjustment.

Research evidence supports each of these assumptions. It is possible to identify children who display many different types of early
problems, and longitudinal studies have documented that children with
such problems are at risk for later more serious difficulties. There are
many situations in which the early onset of problems foreshadows later

more serious problems (e.g., early drug use, externalizing behavioral problems, academic difficulties, depression, sexual activity, and poor peer relationships). There is still much to be learned, however. The precise developmental evolution of many problems is unknown, and we cannot predict exactly which children are most likely to have later problems in the absence of intervention. Nevertheless, the general lesson is that the early appearance of problems does place children at risk for later difficulties. Finally, outcome research from indicated prevention (summarized below) indicates that target groups do show fewer problems following intervention, which would seem to place them at lower risk for future difficulties. In the following discussion, the screening procedures used to identify individuals for intervention are summarized first and then several interventions are described.

Screening Procedures

Screening procedures vary in secondary prevention because different methods are useful for identifying different target problems. Children with externalizing problems such as noncompliance, hyperactivity, or aggression are most commonly identified using teacher and parent rating scales. Self-report instruments are most frequently used to identify youth who are depressed, anxious, or who have low self-esteem. Peer sociometric procedures are used to identify children with poor peer relationships such as those who are social isolates or who are actively rejected by their peers. Other screening procedures that have been used include examining school records to locate children with academic or behavioral problems, and advertising a new program and soliciting referrals from teachers or community agencies (Durlak, 1995).

Many programs have used a multistage, multimethod screening process to identify those in need of intervention. Typically, one method is used in the first stage to screen the entire population of interest and criteria are established to determine those needing further evaluation. For instance, teachers may be asked to complete a brief rating scale on all children in their classes, and those receiving ratings above some predetermined cutoff score are further evaluated. The second stage of evaluation may include behavioral observations, interviews conducted with teachers, parents, or the children themselves, or the administration of some psychological tests to the child. Sometimes, a third evaluation stage is conducted that involves only individuals who meet the criteria established for the second stage of screening. In other words, the size of the population who is evaluated becomes successively smaller over time, until those considered most appropriate for the intervention are selected. Mulitstage screening has been particularly effective in identifying depressed schoolchildren (e.g., Clarke et al., 1995)

Early forms of maladjustment must be identified carefully for at least three reasons. First, all methods of assessing child and adolescent problems are imperfect, so preventionists must check the accuracy of their screening procedures in each setting. Second, a balance must be struck between overidentifying and underidentifying early problems. This issue is often discussed in terms of an assessment procedure's classification or hit rate. That is, does the procedure do a good job of ruling out children who do not have problems (called true negatives), while at the same time accurately identifying those with difficulties (true positives) This issue is very important from a practical standpoint. On the one hand, because only some in the population are eventually singled out for treatment, the child's need for the intervention must be confirmed. On the other hand, there is the possibility that screening for problems may stigmatize selected participants. However, problems must be identified because they can be addressed. Fortunately, secondary prevention programs seldom produce negative effects (Durlak & Wells, 1997b). Therefore, as long as preventionists have confidence in their ability to detect early problems that predict later dysfunction, there is probably greater risk in excluding than including potential program participants.

Third, since many child problems go untreated, it is likely that screening procedures will identify at least a few children who already have serious problems that are more appropriate for therapy than prevention. Preventionists should anticipate this possibility and have a mechanism in place to help such children, for example, arrangements with treatment agencies to receive referrals.

The Legacy of the Primary Mental Health Project

Without a doubt, the group most responsible for promoting the practice of indicated (secondary) prevention is the staff of the Primary Mental Health Project (PMHP), a school-based intervention project headed by Emory Cowen at the University of Rochester. PMHP staff have been active on several fronts. Starting in 1957, they were the first to demonstrate through a series of empirical studies that secondary prevention leads to improved adjustment and that schools are willing to support successful programs. One of the many outcome studies conducted by PMHP is summarized in Table 2.1.

During the 1970s, PMHP actively disseminated the results of their work through workshops, regional dissemination centers connected to

Table 2.1. Representative School-Based Secondary Prevention Programs

| Study | Target groups and problems | Major outcomes | |
		Post	Follow-up findings
Clarke et al. (1995)	Depressed adolescents	—	17 months: fewer diagnosed with mood disorders
Oden & Asher (1977)	Grade 3 and 4; low peer status	Improved peer status	1 year: same as post
Durlak (1977)	Grades 1–3; acting-out & shy–withdrawn problems	Fewer problems	7 months: same as post
Rickel & Lampi (1981)	Preschoolers; cognitive and behavior problems	Improved cognitive and behavioral adjustment	2 years: same as post
Lorion, Caldwell, & Cowen (1976)	Grades 1–3; acting-out and shy–withdrawn problems	Fewer problems	1 year: same as post
Lochman (1992)	Grade 4–6; aggressive and disruptive	Fewer adjustment problems	3 years: less drug use; higher self-esteem; better problem-solving skills
Tremblay et al. (1992)	Grade 1; acting-out problems	—	2 years: fewer with serious problems, more well-adjusted; 6 years: more in regular classes; less delinquent behavior

PMHP, the encouragement of state-level participation in school-based intervention, and consultation to those beginning programs in their community. These dissemination efforts have been very successful. PMHP has influenced the development of early school-based intervention programs operating in about 1500 schools in over 700 school districts around the world, and these schools provide services to at least 50,000 schoolchildren each year (Cowen, Hightower, Pedro-Carroll, Work, & Wyman, 1996).

The original PMHP program has evolved in several ways over the years (Cowen et al., 1996) and its focus on indicated prevention is discussed here. PMHP has promoted a conceptual model of school-based intervention that includes four major components: (1) an emphasis on young children; (2) the development and use of instruments and methods to identify early signs of dysfunction; (3) the use of para-professionals as primary change agents for identified children; and (4) the use of community- and school-based mental health professionals as consultants, trainers, and program evaluators instead of direct service providers.

Brief Review of Indicated Prevention Programs

Many school-based secondary prevention programs have incorporated several features of PMHP's four-pronged conceptual approach while adapting interventions to fit local resources and needs. For example, the PMHP model says nothing about which problems to target and the methods used to resolve them. Investigators have focused on many different types of problems such as depression or anxiety, poor peer relations, behavioral problems of all types, and children with a combination of behavioral and learning difficulties. Teachers, undergraduate and graduate college students, housewives, classroom peers, and mental health professionals have been used as change agents and several different treatment techniques have been used (Durlak, 1995).

Durlak and Wells (1997b) have reviewed the characteristics and outcomes of 130 published and unpublished secondary prevention programs. Program outcomes in the form of mean effect sizes are presented in Fig. 2.2 and 2.3 and indicate that intervention groups improve signifi-

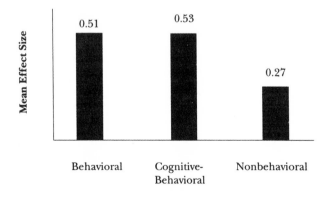

Figure 2.2. Outcomes for different treatments in secondary prevention mental health programs. Data are from Durlak and Wells (1997b).

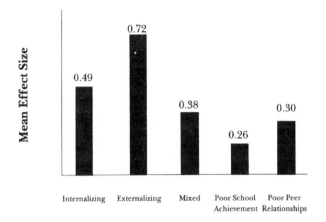

Figure 2.3. Outcomes for different problems targeted in secondary prevention mental health programs. Data are from Durlak and Wells (1997b).

cantly more than controls regardless of their initial problems and what treatment they received. Some treatments and some problems are associated with more change than others, however. For instance, in Fig. 2.2 it can be seen that behavioral and cognitive–behavioral treatments were equally successful and almost twice as effective as nonbehavioral treatment in improving children's adjustment.

Figure 2.3 indicates that outcomes also varied as a function of the children's presenting problems. Somewhat surprisingly, children with externalizing problems demonstrated the best outcomes (mean effect size, 0.72). The least amount of change was obtained with children who had academic problems (mean effect size, 0.26), and children with other difficulties achieved intermediate outcomes (mean effect sizes of 0.30, 0.38, and 0.49). The fact that the best outcomes were achieved for children with externalizing problems is encouraging because externalizing problems are typically not very amenable to change through traditional therapeutic efforts (Kazdin, 1996).

In general, the current empirical status of secondary prevention is very similar to that of primary prevention: Data indicate that certain interventions are effective in significantly improving the adjustment of target populations and these findings should encourage more research and practice on such programs.

Program Examples

Table 2.1 summarizes some exemplary school-based secondary prevention programs conducted at the preschool, elementary, or high school level. These programs have targeted various problems such as social isolation, noncompliance, aggression, and shy–withdrawn behaviors. Furthermore, most of the studies listed in Table 2.1 are part of a programmatic series of reports documenting the ability of early intervention to produce durable and practical changes in children's adjustment.

Oden and Asher (1977) selected socially isolated third and fourth grade children by using peer sociometric ratings to determine who had few friends and did not interact very frequently with peers. Target children were coached in various verbal and nonverbal friendship-making skills associated with peer acceptance. These skills involved cooperation (e.g., taking turns and paying attention), communication (e.g., talking and listening to), and being supportive (e.g., offering compliments, smiling). Immediately following coaching, there was a peer play session that gave the children an opportunity to practice their newly learned skills. This intervention was very successful. Coached children showed significant positive increases in peer sociometric ratings that were maintained during a 1-year follow-up.

Rickel and colleagues have conducted secondary prevention at the preschool level (Rickel & Lampi, 1981; Rickel, Smith, & Sharp, 1979). African-American, low-income children were selected on the basis of a preschool social and cognitive development inventory and a teacher-completed behavioral checklist. Children receiving the poorest scores were seen in individual sessions by college undergraduates. The intervention was individually tailored to meet each child's needs in terms of enhancing their social and cognitive development and modifying their typical acting-out or shy–withdrawn behavioral patterns. Treated children displayed significantly more behavioral and cognitive improvement than controls (Rickel et al., 1979), and these gains were maintained at a 2-year follow-up when the children were in first grade (Rickel & Lampi, 1981). Moreover, at follow-up a normal group of well-adjusted peers was added for comparison purposes and the adjustment of the treatment group did not differ significantly from this group.

Another research group has reported success in using cognitive–behavioral treatment techniques to help middle school boys control their aggressive and disruptive behavior (summarized in Lochman, 1992). In this intervention, school counselors and psychology graduate students co-led groups that taught effective methods of behavioral self-control. A primary focus was the management of anger. Children were reinforced for using self-control techniques and learning appropriate interpersonal problem-solving skills. Evaluations of several treatment cohorts have indicated that the intervention improves children's adjustment in several ways. Off-task, disruptive, and aggressive classroom behaviors are decreased and feelings of social competence are enhanced. A 3-year follow-up indicated continuing effects of intervention; compared to untreated controls, treated children had significantly lower levels of drug use (at follow-up, the children were in midadolescence and in high school) and significantly higher levels of self-esteem and better problem-solving skills (Lochman, 1992). In a fashion similar to Rickel and Lampi's (1981) study, a normal comparison group was available at follow-up. The normal youth and previously treated aggressive boys did not differ significantly on the above outcome measures at follow-up, or on self-reported delinquency and rates of disruptive or off-task classroom behavior.

The Social Skills Development Program (SSDP) (Durlak, 1977) has been implemented in four different school districts (in Heidelberg, Germany; Augusta, Georgia; Carbondale, Illinois; and Pittsburgh, Pennsylvania). In each case, treated children have shown significantly better adjustment than untreated controls following intervention, and positive results have been maintained at follow-up. Children in grades 1 to 3 are selected for SSDP based on teacher ratings reflecting acting-out or shy–withdrawn problems; children with different problems are seen together for weekly 45-minute group sessions. SSDP's behaviorally oriented intervention establishes individualized treatment goals for each participating child. Children with externalizing problems are taught how to exercise greater behavioral self-control and interact more appropriately with peers while those with internalizing difficulties (i.e., shy–withdrawn children) were helped to participate more actively in peer groups and to express their feelings and opinions more assertively.

Durlak and Gillespie (1995) evaluated the changes made by individual children participating in SSDP in two studies by comparing the behavior of program children with a randomly selected group of well-adjusting classroom peers before and after intervention. Data based on behavioral observation of peers were used to define the range of normal behavior in each classroom. In both studies, the pretreatment behavior of all program children was beyond normal limits, that is, program children were displaying more inappropriate behavior than their classroom peers. In the first study, the posttreatment behavior of 83% of the program children fell within the normal range. In the second study, the posttreatment classroom behavior of 74% of program children was within normal limits. The results of these two studies suggest that not only can secondary prevention normalize the behavior of at-risk children, but also that most children (74% to 83%) benefit. Figure 2.4 illustrates these findings.

Data from a Canadian project illustrates that school-based intervention for early forms of disruptive behavior can have positive long-term affects on adjustment (Tremblay, Pagani-Kurtz, Masse, Vitaro, & Pihl, 1995; Tremblay et al., 1992). Teacher rating scales assessing various disruptive behaviors such as fighting, oppositionality, and hyperactivity identified a group of over 300 children who were considered at risk for later problems. Treatment and control groups were created to evaluate the impact of a 2-year intervention that included school and home components.

In the home component, parents received a mean of 17 biweekly individual sessions emphasizing behavioral principles of child management. While parent sessions were occurring, children also received social skills training at school. In these sessions, children were taught friendship-making skills and self-control procedures related to following rules and dealing with anger and other upsetting feelings.

The intervention had a substantial positive impact on children's later social and academic development. For instance, data gathered from peers, teachers, and school records 3 years later were pooled to

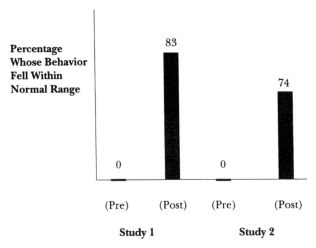

Figure 2.4. Results of two studies reflecting the percentage of program children whose classroom behavior was within normal limits before and after participating in a school-based prevention program. Data are from Durlak and Gillespie (1995).

place each child into one of three outcome categories reflecting their overall school adjustment: well-adjusted, minor problems, and serious difficulties. Only 19% of the control group but 29% of the treated group were considered to be well-adjusted; 50% of the treated group had minor problems compared to 37% of the controls, and the control group contained twice as many children with serious difficulties as the treated group (44% vs. 22%, respectively). These results are important since they suggest that intervention not only reduced the incidence of problems, but also increased the proportion of well-adjusted youth.

A 6-year follow-up study indicated that by age 15, approximately 20% more of the treated group were in age-appropriate regular school classes (Tremblay et al., 1995). Teacher ratings did not indicate any significant treatment versus control group differences in the adolescents' disruptive classroom behavior, but the treatment group did report significantly less delinquent behavior related to drug use, vandalism, and stealing than controls.

In discussing their 6-year follow-up data, Tremblay et al. (1995) suggested that booster sessions be provided in the last year of elementary school and again during the early high school years to help youth prepare for the difficult transition into high school. The need for booster sessions has also been stressed in drug education as a way to promote long-term change (see Chapter 4), and booster sessions have been successfully used in other secondary prevention programs (Lochman, 1992).

Another research group targeted adolescents whose elevated levels of depressive symptomatology suggested risk for eventual clinical depression (Clarke et al., 1995). Students participated in a 15-session cognitive group intervention that targeted such influences on depression as negative cognitions and stressful events. Outcome data covering a 17-month follow-up period indicated significant differences in the proportion of treatment and control adolescents diagnosed as suffering from either major depression or dysthymia (14.5% vs. 25.7%, respectively, over time). In other words, the later rate of clinical mood disorders was 56% lower in the experimental group.

A Community-Based Study

Forehand and colleagues have conducted an impressive series of investigations (summarized in Forehand & Long, 1988; McMahon & Forehand, 1984) on the secondary prevention of externalizing problems. Whereas most secondary prevention programs have been conducted in schools, this project occurred in a community clinic; it deserves special

attention because of the rigor of its evaluation procedures and its positive results.

The Forehand group targeted preschool children demonstrating
noncompliance or more serious acting-out behaviors, because such behaviors in young children predict to later more serious acting-out problems. Operating from a psychology clinic at the University of Georgia,
Forehand and associates solicited referrals from physicians, preschools,
and social agencies. The intervention consisted of a behaviorally oriented parent training program designed to help parents identify and
attend to appropriate child behaviors and the use of appropriate com-
mands and time-out techniques to decrease noncompliant behaviors.
Subsequent studies have added treatment components to address maternal depression and marital communication problems when such problems are present.

In contrast to a typical treatment approach in which all participants
receive all aspects of the intervention in a predetermined time sequence
(e.g., once a week for 10 weeks), participants proceed through the Georgia program at their own pace based on how much time they need to
acquire different parenting skills. Nevertheless, length of treatment averaged only 9 sessions with a range of 5 to 12 sessions. Families in all
socioeconomic groups have successfully completed treatment.

Results indicate that parents can learn child-rearing skills in a brief
period of time and that the acquisition of these skills is related to
significant behavioral improvement in their children. Treated children
demonstrate less noncompliant and more appropriate social behaviors,
and these gains have generalized to home and school settings. The two
most impressive findings from this intervention from a preventive perspective, however, are the social significance of outcomes and their
durability. For example, before intervention, treated children were
found to differ significantly from matched comparison groups of normal
children in their levels of inappropriate behavior; following intervention these differences have disappeared and, in general, have been
maintained at follow-up periods of up to 7½ years. The long-term impact of intervention was examined carefully and thoroughly by search-
ing for adjustment differences between treated and normal comparison
groups in terms of behavioral problems, family relationships, prosocial
behaviors, and levels of school achievement.

SUMMARY

Findings from over 300 controlled outcome studies clearly support
the value of both primary and indicated (secondary) prevention mental

health programs for children and adolescents. In most primary prevention studies, participants have displayed reduced problems and increased competencies; in indicated prevention, early subclinical-level problems have been significantly reduced.

Several examples also suggest that the impact of intervention is durable over time and that prevention produces socially and clinically meaningful changes in children's and adolescents' lives. For instance, it is possible to improve psychological and academic functioning and to reduce the future rates of serious problems such as aggression, depression, vandalism, and delinquency through preventive intervention. In other cases, the level of adjustment of target populations initially at risk for various negative outcomes is later found to be comparable to well-adjusted peer groups following intervention.

Several issues need clarification in the next generation of research. Which factors account for program success? Who profits the most and least from intervention? How well can programs be modified to fit different settings and populations? Nevertheless, extensive empirical data support the value of preventive mental health programs for children and adolescents.

3

Prevention of Learning Problems

EXTENT OF CHILDREN'S LEARNING PROBLEMS

Data drawn from several sources (Dryfoos, 1990; Murphy, 1990; Terman, Larner, Stevenson, & Behrman, 1996; United States Department of Education, 1992) can be pooled to indicate the nature and extent of children's learning problems. There are approximately 2.1 million school children (5%) who have a documented learning disability and 1.2 million (3%) who have developmental disabilities (i.e., mental retardation). On a nation-wide basis, the average writing proficiency of students in the fourth and eighth grades is at less than a minimal level of competency. More than 80% of students in 4th, 10th, and 12th grades demonstrate less than adequate mathematical achievement. One out of every three children experiences significant problems in learning to read, and up to 18% of high school seniors read at least 4 years below grade level. About one out of every five students repeats at least one grade between kindergarten and eighth grade; the annual high school dropout rate is 25%.

Studies have indicated that 80% of young people are unable to summarize adequately the main point of a newspaper article, interpret a bus schedule, or calculate the correct change from a restaurant bill. One half of 13-year-olds do not understand basic aspects of science; almost one half of 17-year-olds cannot perform moderately complex mathematical procedures that are commonly taught 3 to 4 years earlier in junior high school, such as finding an average or interpreting a graph.

Finally, it has been estimated that businesses in the United States spend $25 billion dollars a year training their employees in basic writing, reading, and reasoning skills that they should have learned in school.

Several of the above problems are more serious for certain groups and in certain locales. For instance, school dropout rates for members of minority populations reach 60% or more in some inner-city schools, and up to 40% of minority youth may be functionally illiterate.

In addition to any learning deficits that are present, low expectations and educational standards often undermine young people's potential. For instance, more than one fourth of all public schoolchildren are not being taught appropriate grade-level mathematics material, that is, fourth or fifth grade concepts are being taught in sixth grade (Mac Iver, Reuman, & Main, 1995). This is so despite a growing belief that many children can perform above grade level if given sufficient opportunity and instruction. In summary, there is a need not only to prevent serious learning problems, but also to help youth achieve their full a potential.

Is it realistic to believe that children's learning problems can be prevented and their academic performance significantly enhanced? The answer is "yes." The task is by no means easy, but there is growing evidence that preventive interventions can produce lasting and important positive changes in children's academic functioning. This chapter reviews what is known to date about how to accomplish this task.

FACTORS AFFECTING LEARNING

Many different theories have been advanced to account for learning problems. Early theories tended to view individual factors as most important, including innate intellectual level, motivation, physical health, and emotional conflicts. Contemporary theories, however, postulate that except for the most severe physical or genetic conditions, almost all children can achieve basic proficiency in core academic subjects, and their failure to do so results from the way learning is promoted at school and at home (Lloyd & De Bettencourt, 1986; Walberg, 1984). As a result, partnerships between school and home seem the best way to improve children's learning. Individual factors such as motivation, persistence, and good work habits are not discounted, but are believed to be under considerable environmental influence. Social problems such as crime, violence, and poor employment prospects, and personal and family problems and stress make the task of creating optimal learning environments more difficult, but not impossible.

IMPORTANCE OF EARLY INTERVENTION

Early intervention is critical for the effective prevention of learning problems. Early intervention refers to the preschool years or the first few elementary grades, depending on the situation. Most children do not outgrow their learning problems. Once children demonstrate learning difficulties, they are often unable to catch up to their peers through regular classroom instruction. In many cases, their problems worsen over time, and it becomes more and more difficult to help them master academic tasks. In elementary school the best predictor of future academic performance is current academic performance. As a result, children with early academic problems are at risk for later problems as well.

Before the child reaches elementary school, however, the best overall predictor of academic performance is the family's socioeconomic level. Children from low income households are at greatest risk to demonstrate early learning problems, which, in turn, places them at risk for later problems as well. More than a quarter of all children under age 3 live in poverty (Children's Defense Fund, 1995), and are academically at risk.

The above findings lay the groundwork for the timing of preventive interventions. To prevent later learning problems, intervention during the early elementary school grades is essential; but for those at highest risk (children from poor families), interventions must usually occur before first grade to prepare children for formal schooling. The next two sections discuss programs at these two time periods, beginning first with interventions occurring before elementary school.

EARLY CHILDHOOD PROGRAMS

Programs occurring during infancy, toddlerhood, and the preschool years are generally labeled early childhood education, although a formal educational program may be only one component of these interventions. Some programs even begin during the mother's pregnancy to increase the odds of a healthy birth and delivery, because physical health influences cognitive development.

The Legacy of Head Start

Probably the best-known early childhood program is Head Start, begun during the 1960s as part of President Lyndon Johnson's "War on Poverty." The central idea behind Head Start was to help preschool low-income children prepare for elementary school by stimulating their cognitive and social development. Many Head Start programs did significantly improve children's academic and social development, and in many cases those at greatest risk profited the most (Sylva, 1994). Unfortunately, follow-up studies indicated that many of the gains made from Head Start tended to diminish over time. Many Head Start programs began as brief 8-week summer interventions for 4- and 5-year old children. In retrospect, most educators would agree that the main drawback to Head Start was not that early intervention did not work, but that intervention was neither early nor intensive enough to produce sustained effects. Subsequent research has confirmed that earlier and longer interventions are needed to achieve lasting effects.

Barnett (1990) evaluated 14 early childhood programs that had collected relatively long-term follow-up data on three important indices of children's later school performance: retention in grade, placement in special education, and high school graduation rates. These early childhood programs represented both community- and home-based interventions for infants, toddlers, and preschoolers; parents participated actively in many of these programs. Figure 3.1 summarizes the long-term educational outcomes for experimental and control children. The average follow-up period was 9 years (range from 4 to 14 years).

Overall, 33% fewer children were ever retained in grade (26% vs. 39%), 48% fewer were ever placed in special education (12% vs. 23%), and 24% more students eventually graduated from high school (63% vs. 51%). These are substantial differences, although early intervention did not completely eradicate children's learning problems. Further inspection of the data from each individual study indicates that the experimental group was superior to the control group on every comparison, although some differences were of small magnitude. The consistency in outcomes across so many well-done studies conducted by independent investigators using a variety of intervention procedures, community settings, and populations offers strong evidence for the value of early childhood education.

Commenting on the positive and substantial long-term impact produced by early childhood programs, Barnett (1995) has noted:

> These effects are large enough and persistent enough to make a meaningful difference in the lives of children from low-income families: for many children, preschool programs can mean the difference between failing and passing, regular or special education, staying out of trouble or becoming involved in crime and delinquency, dropping out or graduating from high school. (p. 43)

Others have also reviewed additional early childhood programs and reached the same positive conclusion: Early preventive intervention

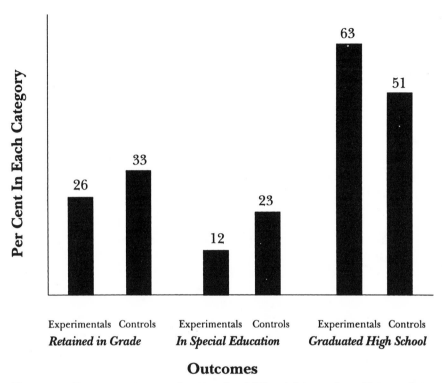

Outcomes

Figure 3.1. Long-term outcomes for 14 early childhood interventions. Data are from Barnett (1990).

can have lasting positive benefits on children's later academic performance (Boocock, 1995; Slavin, Karweit, & Wasik, 1994).

Program Examples

The Perry Preschool Program (PPP) has become one of the most famous early childhood programs because of the broad range of its positive outcomes (Schweinhart & Weikart, 1988). PPP was an intensive 2-year intervention for low-income families that combined a 5-day/week preschool curriculum for 3- and 4-year-old children with a home-visiting program. Preschool teachers made weekly home visits to help parents promote their child's social and cognitive development in coordination with the preschool curriculum. Teachers also helped parents secure needed medical and social services for their families. A 14-year follow-up indicated that the experimental children were superior to controls on many outcomes including grades, grade retentions, time spent in special education, rates of mental retardation (15% vs. 35%), and the proportion of students who graduated from high school (67% vs. 49%). Positive effects also included such social and vocational outcomes as later arrest rates (31% vs. 51%), employment status (50% vs. 32%), and post-high school education (38% vs. 21%). Economic evaluations have indicated that PPP is very cost-effective, returning approximately $8 dollars in benefits for every dollar spent (see Chapter 8).

One of the most dramatic findings from PPP was the 39% reduction in the number of adolescents who were ever arrested. Long-term reductions in serious acting-out behavior have also been obtained for other early childhood programs (Yoshikawa, 1995). These data support the rather startling conclusion that one way to prevent delinquency is through early childhood intervention.

Another successful early childhood program has been the Abecedarian Project, whose evaluation illustrates the importance of intensity and timing in early intervention (Horacek, Ramey, Campbell, Hoffmann, & Fletcher, 1987). Three experimental cohorts and an untreated control group were studied over time. Experimental group 1 received an intensive early intervention program lasting from birth to age 5; experimental group 2 received this early intervention plus a later less-intensive program in elementary school; and experimental group 3 received only the later less-intensive elementary program. Analyses suggested a direct relationship between school success and the timing and intensity of the intervention. The percentage of children who had repeated a grade by the end of third grade was 50% for the control group, 38% for group 3 (who had only received the later elementary program), 29% for group 1 (early intensive program only), but only 16% for those in group 2, who had received both the early and later programs. Analyses of school grades reflected a similar pattern of findings.

Additional follow-up was conducted when the children were approximately 15 years old (Campbell & Ramey, 1995). These data indicated that experimental group 3 (elementary school intervention only) tended not to differ from the untreated controls on most outcomes, but that both groups receiving the preschool intervention (experimental groups 1 and 2) continued to do well. In fact, after 10 years in school, children in the latter two groups had significantly higher reading and math test scores and were almost four times less likely to be placed in special education programs than the untreated controls (12% vs. 47%, respectively). The Abecedarian Project thus joins PPP as a very carefully evaluated early intervention whose practical results have been sustained into adolescence.

The loss of effect for the elementary school intervention group over time led investigators from the Abecedarian Project to conclude: "... those who plan interventions for poor children should be aware that elementary school programs may have less impact on the children's academic performance than would programs begun earlier in the life span" (Campbell & Ramey, 1995, p. 769).

Studies done outside the United States also support the long-term impact of early intervention. Boocock (1995) evaluated research on early childhood programs conducted in 13 countries (Australia, Canada, Colombia, France, Germany, India, Ireland, Japan, Singapore, South Korea, Sweden, Turkey, and the United Kingdom). Despite program variations across countries to account for different social and cultural contexts, Boocock (1995) concluded that international research supports the notion that early intervention "... can have strong positive effects on children's school readiness and their subsequent academic performance" (p. 103).

A carefully done, long-term study conducted in Turkey illustrates findings from other countries. The Turkey Early Enrichment Project (Kagitcibasi, 1995) randomly assigned low-income families with young children in Istanbul to experimental and control conditions. Beginning at age 3, children attended a 2-year child care program and their mothers concurrently received systematic training on how to stimulate their child's cognitive and social development at home. Mothers also participated in biweekly group discussions to learn problem-solving and child management skills and received social support from project staff and other mothers.

A follow-up 7 years later when the children were entering early adolescence indicated lasting effects from the intervention across several outcome domains: 86% of the experimental children were still in school compared to 67% of the controls, and the former had earned significantly higher school grades. None in the experimental group (vs. 6% of the controls) had ever experienced any trouble with the law, and the adolescents in the experimental group enjoyed greater personal autonomy and better peer relationships. At follow-up, parents involved in the intervention held higher educational aspirations for their children and reported better parent–child communication and closer and better family relations.

Elements of Successful Interventions

Successful early childhood programs combine several elements, and it is unknown how different features contribute to outcomes. For example, preschool programs vary in their philosophy and approach;

some are highly structured, some emphasize academic or preacademic skills, whereas others focus on play and social development. Specific program features may not be as important as having a well-trained and experienced teaching staff and a low teacher-to-child ratio so that children receive individual attention suited to their developmental needs. Duration and intensity are also important; at least 1 year and preferably 2 or more years of a half-day or full-day program is usually necessary to produce the best results. Furthermore, effective programs offer many services to parents such as assistance in child care and behavioral management, training in how to promote the child's social and cognitive development, social support, and health services. In effect, many programs seek to empower the child's primary caretakers so they can function as effective advocates for themselves and their children.

Importance of School Readiness

One useful concept for understanding the impact of early childhood programs is school readiness, which is a multidimensional construct that refers to the developmental maturation of physical, cognitive, and social skills that enable children to complete an academic curriculum successfully (Lewit & Baker, 1995). Although there is no single definition or criterion, school readiness includes such things as the ability to speak clearly and understandably, to sit still, to take turns and follow instructions, being interested in learning, and being in adequate physical condition to learn (e.g., being healthy and receiving sufficient sleep and nutrition). School readiness exists along a continuum, and children begin elementary school at different levels of school readiness.

On the one hand, data suggest that more than one out of every three children (35%) is not fully ready for school entry (Lewit & Baker, 1995). Many of these children come from low-income households, which is consistent with the fact that such populations are academically at risk. On the other hand, research demonstrates quite clearly that school readiness can be enhanced through intervention. A formal preschool program to foster children's social and cognitive development is one obvious component to such interventions, but parental behaviors are also important.

In fact, research is beginning to suggest that parental activities such as the learning environment they create at home and their ability to promote social skills needed for effective learning such as self-control and cooperation are significant influences on school readiness and can be more important than the parents' educational and socioeconomic level (Morrison, Griffith, Williamson, & Hardway, 1995). As a result, a majority of successful early childhood programs have combined school and home interventions. In summary, successful early childhood programs thus demonstrate how partnerships between school and home foster children's academic development.

INTERVENTIONS AT THE ELEMENTARY LEVEL

Tutoring

One of the oldest and most basic educational strategies has emerged as one of the most successful preventive interventions at the elementary school level: tutoring. Several investigators have independently concluded that well-implemented tutoring programs are effective in improving academic performance, particularly for at-risk students (Cohen, Kulik & Kulik, 1982; Fantuzzo, King, & Heller, 1992; Greenwood, Carta, & Hall, 1988; Slavin et al., 1994). Following a careful review of preventive programs, Slavin et al. (1994) stated that "One-on-one tutoring is the most effective form of instruction known" (p. 178).

There is particular value in peer tutoring, since research suggests that student tutors benefit socially and academically from the tutoring role. In some cases, tutors have gained more than the students they are tutoring (Cohen et al., 1982; Greenwood et al., 1988). In addition to academic gains, tutoring has also produced significant improvements in social and behavioral adjustment such as more positive attitudes toward school, better peer relations, decreases in disruptive behavior, and improved self-concepts (see Fantuzzo et al., 1992; Greenwood et al., 1988).

Two very successful peer tutoring programs that have several features in common are Reciprocal Peer Tutoring (RPT) (Fantuzzo et al., 1992) and Classwide Peer Tutoring (CWPT) (Greenwood, Delquadri, & Hall, 1989). Each program has been used extensively with academically at-risk elementary school children. In each approach, students from the same class are paired for tutoring sessions and alternate being tutors and tutees; students are rewarded for their academic progress.

Greenwood et al. (1989) conducted an extensive, 4-year longitudinal study of CWPT. Over 400 students and 94 teachers from grades 1 to 4 in 25 schools participated. CWPT was implemented at various times during the children's first 4 years in school. The academic achievement of tutored children from low-socioeconomic status (SES) families was compared to two groups: (1) an untutored control group from similar low-SES homes; and, (2) children from high-SES families who eventually served as a local standard for good academic performance. At the end of 4 years, not only did tutored children significantly outperform low-SES controls in reading, mathematics, and language on standardized achievement tests, but their performance also did not differ significantly from the high-SES group who were doing well in school.

Tutoring is a good preventive intervention because of its flexibility. Tutoring can be used as either a primary or secondary (indicated) prevention strategy; it can be implemented in a variety of settings (e.g., in and outside the classroom or at home) and it can be conducted by several different change agents (peers, teachers, teacher aides, parents, or college undergraduates). Most importantly, the intensity and duration of tutoring can be varied to suit student needs. The latter features are very important, because some students will need more tutoring than others in some subjects or need assistance in multiple subjects.

Two cautions must be expressed relative to tutoring programs. First, most tutoring has focused on the acquisition of basic skills, so its value in promoting higher-order cognitive and reasoning skills is unknown. Second, tutoring programs are not easy interventions to administer. Good tutor training and monitoring of a tutor's performance are essential; programs that are not effectively implemented achieve fewer benefits (Greenwood, Terry, Arreaga-Mayer, & Finney, 1992).

Success for All

Success for All (SFA) is a unique program that spans the preschool and early elementary school period in a comprehensive approach at prevention and early intervention. It is based on the premise "... that the school must *relentlessly continue with every child until that child is succeeding*" (Slavin et al., 1994, p. 176, italics are the authors).

SFA combines several features that characterize successful academic interventions: it is intensive, it begins early with a preschool program, it involves parents, and it emphasizes tutoring in the early elementary grades. SFA began in 1986 in the Baltimore schools and has spread to several school districts across the country. The program varies depending on local resources, but SFA typically begins with a half-day preschool and kindergarten program that emphasizes both academic readiness and social development. When the child reaches first grade, daily one-on-one tutoring in reading occurs in sessions conducted by paid adult tutors. Additional tutoring is offered to those in need. The adult tutors also assist the regular classroom teacher during the day's 90-minute classroom reading periods. A writing–arts program based primarily on cooperative learning principles is introduced beginning in second grade. Finally, family support teams are created at each SFA school; these teams offer social support and educational services to parents, monitor the school attendance and performance of individual children, and work with teachers or parents to promote child learning.

SFA has been very effective. One analysis combined 43 experimental cohorts of students from grades 1 to 3 drawn from eight schools in four cities (Slavin et al., 1994). The schools served racially and ethnically diverse low-income populations and were located in rural and inner-city settings. In terms of reading achievement, SFA students significantly outperformed controls at all grade levels, and the longer students had participated in SFA, the more they benefited. Students most at risk based on their initial levels of reading skills demonstrated nearly twice the overall benefit of other students. Furthermore, there were many more SFA students with high levels of achievement and many fewer with poor levels. Compared to matched controls, there were 49.5% more SFA students reading 1 year or more above grade level and 41% fewer who were reading 1 year or more below grade level. Finally, control students were 50% more likely than SFA students to be placed in special education classes. Slavin et al. (1994) have concluded that various outcome studies of SFA indicate it is possible to "... ensure the school success of the majority of disadvantaged at-risk students" (p. 216).

INDICATED PREVENTION

Indicated prevention occurs after children have demonstrated some early learning problems but before their difficulties have become very serious. Unfortunately, many indicated preventive interventions for young schoolchildren (in educational parlance, compensatory or remedial education programs) are of dubious value (see Slavin et al., 1989). The main problem appears to be that most of these programs are neither intensive nor extensive enough to help children catch up to their peers.

Slavin et al. (1989) did identify, however, approximately two dozen indicated prevention programs that were successful in significantly improving young children's reading achievement. Several different types of programs were effective. There were some one-on-one tutoring programs, some emphasizing computer-assisted instruction, and some emphasizing cooperative learning. In cooperative learning, students with different ability levels are assigned to teams and they work together to help each other master assigned materials. The largest number of effective programs fell under the rubric of continuous progress programs. In these programs, student progress is carefully monitored as they proceed step by step through a hierarchy of specific learning tasks. DISTAR is one example of a continuous learning program.

In DISTAR, teachers use very specific teaching techniques with small groups of students of equal ability. DISTAR emphasizes direct teacher instruction, fast pacing, and constant practice and repetition to achieve mastery. DISTAR has been used in several different school districts across the country, and although some educators do not like the highly structured, scripted lessons, DISTAR produces good results. DISTAR students typically display significantly higher achievement than control students in such subjects as reading, mathematics, and language, and they maintain these gains up to 3 years after intervention (Becker & Carnine, 1980). DISTAR students also show increased levels of self-esteem. Most importantly, following intervention, DISTAR students approach or exceed national norms on most academic measures. Although normative performance does slip for some cohorts over time (Becker & Gersten, 1982), in some cases impressive long-term outcomes have been achieved. In one program, high school graduation rates were 62% higher for inner-city students initially exposed to DISTAR than for controls (Meyer, 1984).

Characteristics of Effective Interventions

Successful primary and indicated prevention programs at the elementary school level differ in terms of specific materials, curricula, and various program practices. Nevertheless, effective programs tend to use eight basic pedagogic principles:

1. Structure the intervention carefully using a step-by-step process to achieve specific goals. Those occupying teaching roles, (teachers, aides, parents, or peers) must know what to do and when.
2. Directly teach students what you want them to learn; avoid focusing on indirect methods to enhance performance such as training in perceptual or motor processes. These indirect approaches are not effective in increasing academic achievement.
3. Devote as much time as possible to academic instruction; in general, greater amounts of academic learning time promote higher levels of achievement.
4. Provide help quickly whenever signs of difficulty appear.
5. Present material suited to students' ability levels; the material should be challenging, but not so difficult that mastery is impossible.

6. Monitor student progress frequently and make adjustments in the pacing and level of instruction to account for individual learning styles and the need for more practice and repetition.
7. Reinforce students for both effort and product.
8. Provide instruction that is intensive and of sufficient duration to insure mastery of target skills.

What is striking about these eight principles is that they are generally consistent with what is known about effective teaching practices in the regular school classroom (Brophy, 1986). In other words, teachers do not have to learn a new set of pedagogic practices and philosophies to participate in preventive programs. Effective teaching techniques seem to work for all types of students.

CLASSROOM AND SCHOOL FACTORS

Learning does not take place in a vacuum and it is also important to examine and perhaps change the broader social context in which academic instruction occurs. The next two sections describe efforts to modify the classroom and entire school in order to promote students' academic achievement and prevent problems.

Classroom Environments

Measures that assess the social environment or climate of the classroom usually focus on three main environmental dimensions: (1) interpersonal relationships (e.g., are those in the setting involved with and supportive of each other?); (2) goal orientation (e.g., are activities in the setting centered on accomplishing specific objectives?); and (3) system maintenance and change (e.g., is the setting structured and well-organized?). In general, student academic achievement, peer relations, and attitudes toward school are enhanced in environments that are supportive, well-organized, and goal-directed (see Fraser & Walberg, 1991).

Changing Classroom Environments

One successful example of a preventive intervention at the level of the classroom involves proactive classroom management (PCM). PCM has three central features: (1) a focus on preventing inappropriate behaviors; (2) a recognition of the inseparability of students' personal and social behavior and their learning activities; and (3) an emphasis on classroom-level management rather than attention to only a few individuals (Gettinger, 1988),

PCM is a complicated proactive method of classroom organization and management that helps teachers create a well-ordered and supportive learning environment. Teachers learn how to communicate clearly to their students about what is expected, how student performance will be monitored and evaluated, and what consequences are attached to different levels of performance. On a day-by-day basis, teachers adept at PCM know how to pace instruction to match student progress, carefully monitor student behavior, help students who are having difficulty, and redirect students who are off-task or off-track. In effect, the successful use of PCM would create the type of classroom environment that research indicates is conducive to student growth and productivity (that is, a supportive and well-organized class with a clear academic focus).

Evertson and colleagues (Evertson, 1985; Evertson, Emmer, Sanford, & Clements, 1983) have demonstrated that: (1) both elementary and secondary school teachers can develop PCM skills; (2) local school administrators can be used to train and supervise teachers in PCM techniques, thus increasing the possibility of transporting this intervention into many schools; and, most important, (3) the use of PCM results in significant reductions in student misbehavior and significant increases in on-task behaviors. PCM is now being incorporated into school-based preventive programs (e.g., Hawkins et al., 1991).

Effective Schools

There is a large literature on effective schools, in growing recognition of the fact that schools do make a difference in students' lives. Schools have effects beyond what would be predicted based on their financial resources, the experience level or degrees of the staff, and students' initial ability levels. In some cases, the type of school a child attends is five times more important than the student's family or socioeconomic background (Sylva, 1994).

Although the notion of effective schools has received substantial empirical support, exactly why schools are successful and which features are most important are less clear. It is likely that numerous factors interact. Those most frequently associated with effective schools are: (1) a primary emphasis on the acquisition of basic skills coupled with high expectations for student achievement; (2) strong leadership and administrative support; (3) a well-organized, safe environment that encourages learning; (4) frequent monitoring of student progress and consistent reinforcement of good performance; (5) a shared sense of purpose and values among staff that fosters collaboration, mutual support, and positive relationships between teachers and students; (6) a schoolwide program of staff development; and (7) a high level of parent participation in their children's school life. The last two characteristics deserve specific discussion because they are frequently overlooked or misunderstood.

Staff Development

Teaching is in large part a lonely and stressful occupation, and many teacher education programs do not prepare their students adequately for the realities of the classroom. At least a third of teachers leave the profession within 7 years (Fullan, 1992), while an unknown proportion of those who remain on the job are affected by stress or burnout that lessens their productivity.

Being a good teacher requires a lifelong commitment to learning in order to accommodate to new curricula, changing student bodies, and social and political pressures affecting schools. Therefore, schools must provide meaningful opportunities for teachers' personal and professional growth. Part of staff development involves giving teachers some decision-making input into changing school practices and policies and developing mechanisms for teachers to support and help each other. Sarason (1993) has wisely observed: "If conditions for productive growth do not exist for teachers, they cannot create and sustain those conditions for students" (pp. 256–257). Several good sources offer helpful comments about improving working conditions for teachers (Fullan, 1992; Sarason, 1993).

Parent Participation

Research has confirmed that the more parents participate in their children's education, the higher their children's level of achievement, a finding that holds across all socioeconomic, ethnic, or racial groups. In fact, the evidence for the value of parental involvement "... is as impressive as any in the field of educational change" (Fullan, 1992, p. 228). At the same time, high levels of parent participation should be considered a characteristic of effective schools because it is up to the schools to encourage and support parents' participation. School practices and policies appear to be the most important variable influencing parents' level of participation (Epstein, 1990). If the school does not make a conscientious effort to engage all parents, then only some will become involved, and most of these are likely to come from the ranks of those with higher levels of education and income. Most parents, however, want to be involved in their child's education and want to learn how they can help. Furthermore, parents can benefit from their participation by becoming more sensitive to their children's needs and developing greater self-confidence in their parenting abilities.

Parent involvement takes many forms such as monitoring their children's school performance and behavior and staying in contact with teachers, tutoring their children at home if necessary, assisting in the school's social and recreational activities, and being active in school governance and decision making. There are many examples in the literature of how increasing parental involvement enhances children's school functioning, confirming the importance of an effective working relationship between schools and families (Christenson, Rounds, & Gorney, 1992; Epstein, 1990). The program descriptions below illustrate some ways in which parents have been successfully involved in their children's education as part of schoolwide efforts at reorganization and improvement.

Making Schools More Effective

Introducing organizational or systemic changes in schools to make them more effective is complicated and time consuming. No single approach will work in all situations, since schools vary in their personnel, resources, leadership, and student bodies. The three examples below represent different techniques used in improving schools.

One effort to develop more effective schools is Project Achieve, an attempt at schoolwide reform designed to enhance children's academic performance and social adjustment (Knoff & Batsche, 1995). Project Achieve has four major components: (1) training teachers in more effective teaching practices and classroom management skills; (2) involving parents more actively in their children's schoolwork; (3) improving parental child-rearing skills; and (4) promoting children's social skill development, particularly in the areas of self-control.

Strategic planning sessions involving all school staff produce a set of joint goals and agreed-upon procedures to meet these goals. As plans are put into motion, parents learn positive behavior management approaches to work with their own children at home and are also trained as academic tutors. Teachers learn new classroom techniques through in-service team teaching programs and receive ongoing consultation and guidance from teachers or other school staff.

Results for Project Achieve have been impressive. Over a 5-year period in one elementary school district serving racially and ethnically diverse low-income families, placements in special education class-rooms were reduced by 67%, grade retentions declined by 90%, total disciplinary referrals declined by 28%, and school suspensions declined by 64%. Comparisons between program and control schools indicated that students in Project Achieve were more than three times less likely to be placed in special education classes and more than five times less likely to repeat a grade. Standardized achievement test data indicated that 17.8% more Project Achieve students were performing at or above grade level.

The Yale–New Haven Project (Comer, 1985) created a new administrative and decision-making school structure. Teachers, administrators, parents, and community-based mental health professionals collaborated to govern the school, set policies, and monitor new programs. This program thus represents the highest level of parent involvement in their children's school life, since parents sat on several governing boards and school committees. The general goal of this intervention was to develop programs and curricula that would create a positive school climate, good relationships between teachers and students, and an effective working partnership between the school and families. Various programs were initiated to promote students' academic, social, and recreational development. The project began in two inner-city schools serving primarily low-income African-American families. Although the two schools had historically low levels of achievement and high rates of behavior and attendance problems over time, the students' academic performance rose to near the top of city rankings, while serious behavioral and attendance problems were virtually eliminated. A 3-year follow-up indicated students were performing at grade level in most of their subjects and were approximately 2 years ahead of controls; program students also gained significantly in self-confidence and social competencies.

A third illustration of successful school change is the cooperative school (Stevens & Slavin, 1995). Once again, several elements characterized the intervention. The principal and teachers worked collaboratively to make two major changes in academic practices: (1) cooperative learning strategies were introduced for most academic subjects; and (2) children with learning disabilities were mainstreamed into regular classes. Extensive teacher peer coaching was used to increase the quality of implementation. Peer coaching involves opportunities for teachers to observe and give feedback to one another. Teachers with expertise demonstrate new techniques and then observe and give feedback as other teachers use these new methods in their own classrooms. The principal participates by taking over classes for teachers who must leave their class for peer coaching activities. A final element of the cooperative school was parent involvement. Principals and teachers encouraged parents to monitor their children's school progress and to encourage their children to meet the school's educational expectations.

Outcomes were assessed separately for children with learning disabilities, for gifted students, and for the remainder of the student body. Results indicated that all three groups profited compared to students in a control school, and gains were evident in academic achievement, academic self-concepts, and peer relationships. The finding that students in different educational categories profit in multiple ways indicates the value of making schoolwide changes.

Importance of Social Norms and Values

Cross-cultural comparisons indicate that it may be necessary to modify parental educational attitudes and values in the United States in order to enhance students' academic achievement. Stevenson, Chen, and Lee (1993) were interested in identifying some of the factors accounting for the significantly higher achievement in mathematics consistently attained by students in China and Taiwan compared to the United States. The academic differences are striking. Among fifth graders, only 4.1% of Chinese children and 10.1% of Japanese children scored as low as the *average* American child; a similar pattern was found among 10th graders. Basically, these researchers concluded that these achievement differences do not come about because of innate differences in intellectual ability, but because parents and schools in China and Taiwan act in unison to help children attain high goals. For instance, Asian schools are structured so that students are expected to work hard to achieve high standards and students are consistently supported in their progress toward these standards by both teachers and parents. There is much more academic learning time devoted to mathematics in Chinese and Taiwanese schools than in American schools. The curriculum is also more demanding; Asian students are exposed to more difficult subject matter earlier in school than in the United States and are expected to master more mathematical material overall.

There are also striking differences in parental educational practices and attitudes. Despite the relatively poor achievement of their children compared to Asian students, American parents overestimated their childrens' current academic performance. By comparison, American parents also expected less from their children academically; they were much less involved in their child's schoolwork and academic life. Finally, they believed that academic success was much more strongly influenced by innate ability rather than effort. This last finding suggests that American parents are less likely to believe their children could do better if they worked harder and tried to reach higher goals. Under such circumstances, it might be difficult to convince some parents of the importance of individual effort in reaching academic goals.

Good Academic Performance as a Protective Factor

Poor academic performance is associated with a variety of negative outcomes such as various behavioral and psychological problems, poor peer relations, drug use, and delinquency. There is accumulating evidence, however, that good academic performance may serve as a protective factor for these outcomes. For example, there is the dramatic finding from the Perry Preschool Program, a preschool intervention, that improved academic performance was also associated with significant long-term reductions in adolescent acting-out behavior. Similar results have been reported in other programs (Yoshikawa, 1995). Other successful academic programs discussed in this chapter have also produced positive changes in students' disruptive behaviors, self-concept and self-esteem, and peer relations (e.g., Comer, 1985; Fantuzzo et al., 1992; Knoff & Batsche, 1995; Stevens & Slavin, 1995).

Finally, it is probably no coincidence that at least four independent groups of investigators interested in preventing behavioral problems have added academic components to their interventions (Coie & Krehbiel, 1984; Cowen et al., 1996; Hawkins et al., 1991; Jason et al., 1992). Each of these programs has reported positive results. In summary, it is especially important to attend to children's academic needs when planning preventive interventions. Promoting children's academic performance may be one way to protect them against a variety of possible negative outcomes in addition to poor school achievement.

SUMMARY

Several interventions have been able to prevent later learning problems. For instance, the percentage of students who later flunk a grade, are placed in special education, drop out of school, or fail to do well academically has been reduced from 26 to 90%, depending on the study and the specific outcome. Early intervention appears to be critical to the success of such programs. For the more than one quarter of young American children who live in poverty and are at high academic risk, intervention should occur during infancy and the preschool years and should be focused on promoting school readiness—an important bellwether of future academic performance.

For children in elementary school, intensive intervention should begin at the point of school entry to ensure mastery of basic academic skills. Many successful elementary-level programs have followed similar pedagogic principles such as using clear educational objectives, devoting as much time as possible to direct academic instruction, and continual monitoring of student performance, with recurring opportunities for practice and feedback until mastery is achieved.

School quality makes a significant contribution to student achievement, so it may be necessary to make organizational or systemic changes to enhance the learning of all students. Effective schools have high academic standards; create a safe, organized, and supportive learning environment; and are characterized by administrators, teachers, students, and parents working collaboratively to achieve common goals. Effective partnerships between schools and families are also important at all educational levels and for families from all racial, ethnic, and socioeconomic groups. The more parents participate in their children's school life, the higher the level of children's achievement.

Finally, there is growing evidence that good academic performance is a protective factor in young people's lives that can lessen the future likelihood of negative outcomes such as crime and delinquency and various psychological and behavioral problems. The academic needs of target populations should not be overlooked in preventive interventions.

4

Drug Prevention

INTRODUCTION

Drug use is prevalent among young people. In 1994, almost half of all high school students (46%) tried at least one illicit drug, such as marijuana, hallucinogens, cocaine, or stimulants. Furthermore, 80% tried alcohol, 63% cigarettes, and 31% smokeless tobacco. The quantity or level of drug use is also a concern. More than one out of every ten youth (11.2%) are smoking a half a pack of cigarettes or more each day and 28% of seniors have gotten drunk within the past month. Drug use is also occurring at an earlier age. By eighth grade, 50% of students have tried alcohol and half of these students (26%) have gotten drunk at least once; 46% have tried cigarettes, 30% smokeless tobacco, 20% inhalants, 17% marijuana, and more than one third (35%) have tried at least one illicit drug.

> Despite the improvements between 1979 and 1991, it is still true that this nation's secondary school students and young adults show a level of involvement with illicit drugs which is greater than has been documented in any other industrialized nation in the world. Even by longer-term historical standards in this country, these rates remain extremely high. Heavy drinking also remains widespread and troublesome; and certainly the continuing initiation of a large and growing proportion of young people to cigarette smoking is a matter of the greatest public health concern. (Johnston, O'Malley, & Bachman, 1995, p. 27)

In addition, the immoderate or impulsive use of drugs places youth at risk for other problems such as school difficulties, violence and crime, physical injury, and unprotected sexual intercourse, raising the specter of sexually transmitted disease, pregnancy, and AIDS. For instance, between 18 to 50% of youth report drinking in connection with their first sexual experience, and drinking is also associated with the nonuse of contraception (Leigh, Schafer, & Temple, 1995). Alcohol also has been implicated in over 50% of all vehicle crashes resulting in serious injury or death for those under age 21 (Vegega & Klitzner, 1988).

The total costs associated with alcohol and drug abuse are believed to exceed $110 billion each year in the United States (National Commission on Children, 1991). Prevention is extremely important, since treatment for alcohol and drug abuse is generally not very effective and relapse rates are high (Bukstein, 1995; Schinke, Botvin, & Orlandi, 1991).

BRIEF HISTORY OF DRUG INTERVENTIONS

There has been a major transformation in approaches to drug prevention over time. Alcohol was the initial focus of attention. Beginning in the late nineteenth century, efforts were initiated by private groups, churches, and social organizations (e.g., the Women's Christian Temperance Union) to discourage the use of alcohol for religious or moral reasons (Bukstein, 1995). A later reflection of this moral movement against alcohol was Prohibition, legislation enacted in 1919 that outlawed the production and sale of alcoholic beverages in the United States and which was later repealed.[1] There was a reawakening of interest in drug prevention in the early 1960s that was spurred in large part by recognition of increased drug use among young people. It was then that multiple substances began receiving attention: tobacco, alcohol, and illegal drugs such as marijuana, heroin, and hallucinogens.

Many school-based drug prevention programs were initiated during the 1960s and early 1970s. Unfortunately, the general conclusion that emerged from program evaluations conducted in this era was pessimistic. Most programs did not change behavior. The thrust of many early programs was on providing information about drugs, in particular their harmful consequences, based on the belief that such tactics would prevent drug use. We now know these early drug programs were founded on incorrect assumptions. Simply imparting information or scaring young people does not deter them from taking drugs.

A few investigations began appearing, however, suggesting that so-called psychosocial intervention was effective. Psychosocial programs generally target interpersonal and social factors that influence drug use such as peer and adult modeling, peer pressure, and media and community influences. The success of such programs stimulated considerable

[1]Although Prohibition did not eliminate drinking as its proponents had hoped, it did have some positive effects. The US national death rate for cirrhosis dropped 39% while Prohibition was in effect, but rose 222% in the years following its repeal.

additional activity in psychosocial programs. A rapid progression in the
theoretical and methodological sophistication of drug interventions has
occurred within the past few years as investigators have generally confirmed the value of a psychosocial approach to intervention. Several
research teams have reported success in preventing drug use and have
developed methods to increase the long-term impact of interventions, to
export programs for use in multiple sites, and to culturally tailor programs for specific populations. Although there are still several unknowns, there is now a growing body of work that attests to the positive
impact of drug prevention.

SUCCESSFUL DRUG PREVENTION PROGRAMS

Table 4.1 presents details on some outcome studies that are exemplary in terms of their conceptualization, execution, and evaluation.
Although every study does not contain every feature, the investigations
in Table 4.1 are theory-driven, large-scale, randomized field trials involving many schools and children (notice the very large sample sizes),
and care is taken to examine how well the intervention has been implemented, how different participants benefit from the program, and if
program effects endure over time. The follow-up periods range from 2 to
8 years.

The magnitude of change achieved in these studies has been impressive. Comparisons between program and comparison groups indicate that the percentage of students who later smoke has been reduced
by 28 to 39% (Flynn et al., 1994; Perry, Kelder, Murray, & Klepp, 1992;
Vartiainen, Pallonen, McAlister, & Puska, 1990); the percentage who
later use marijuana has been reduced by 18 to 38% (Cheadle et al., 1995;
Johnson et al., 1990); the percentage using alcohol has been reduced by
19 to 45% (Hansen & Graham, 1991; Perry et al., 1996); and the odds of
smoking, drinking immoderately, or using marijuana have been reduced
by 40% or more (Botvin, Baker, Dusenbury, Botvin, & Diaz, 1995). In
other words, interventions have produced socially meaningful changes
in drug behaviors. The programs in Table 4.1 can be divided into skills
training interventions and skills training plus communitywide programs, which are briefly discussed in the next two sections.

Skills Training Programs

Two types of successful skills training programs are resistance skills
programs and the Life Skills Training (LST) program, which focuses on

Table 4.1. Exemplary Drug Prevention Outcome Studies

Study	Sample size/ grade level	Target drug(s)	Emphasis of intervention	Major findings	Follow-up (in months)
Botvin et al. (1995)	3597; grades 5 and 6	Tobacco, alcohol, marijuana	Life skills training	Reduced use for all target drugs	36
Cheadle et al. (1995)	3073; grades 9–12	Alcohol, marijuana, tobacco	School and community program	Reduced alcohol use	
Dielman et al. (1989)	1505; grades 5 and 6	Alcohol	Resistance training	Students with prior use show less alcohol use and misuse	26
Flynn et al. (1994)	5458; grades 4–6	Tobacco	1. Resistance training 2. 1 plus mass media	2 > 1 on cigarette smoking	24
Hansen & Graham (1991)	2135; grade 7	Alcohol, tobacco, marijuana	1. Resistance training 2. Social norms 3. 1 plus 2 4. Information only	2,3 > 1, 4 for all target drugs	None
Johnson et al. (1990)	1607; grades 6 and 7	Tobacco, alcohol, marijuana	School plus community program	Reduced tobacco and marijuana use	36
Perry et al. (1992)	2401; grade 7	Tobacco	School plus community program	Reduced tobacco use	60
Perry et al. (1996)	2351; grades 6–8	Alcohol	School plus community program	Reduced alcohol use	None
Vartiainen et al. (1990)	743; grades 7 and 8	Tobacco	School plus community program	Reduced tobacco use	96

general social skills. Resistance skills (sometimes called refusal skills) programs train children in specific skills useful in resisting social and interpersonal pressures to take drugs. For instance, children learn to communicate their wishes effectively and assert themselves in social situations in which drugs may be offered. A social learning approach is used to teach resistance skills, and training consists of first defining and modeling of the target skills and then practice of the skills in a role-playing situation followed by positive feedback and reinforcement. In some resistance skills programs, children are also taught to detect media portrayals and maneuvers used by advertisers to promote drug use. Peer leaders who do not use drugs are often involved in resistance skills programs and lead or colead program sessions along with teachers or research staff.

LST has a slightly different orientation and focuses on multiple coping and interpersonal skills applicable not only to drugs but also to other personal and social situations. LST trains youth in communication and assertive skills, decision making and goal setting, self-directed behavior change strategies, and cognitive–behavioral coping techniques to deal with anxiety and social pressure. A social learning training approach is also taken in LST programs. LST has been evaluated in more research studies than any other single type of drug program and has consistently been effective (Dusenbury, Botvin, & James-Ortiz, 1990). Furthermore, although initially developed as a school-based intervention, LST has been successfully used in community settings (St. Pierre, Kaltreider, Mark, & Aiken, 1992).

Communitywide Programs

Some programs in Table 4.1 have incorporated skills training school-based programs within broader communitywide interventions. These community programs rest on the premise that an individual-level intervention will not be as effective as one that also involves parents, the media, community agencies, and businesses. Positive changes occurring throughout the community should provide models, social norms, supports, and reinforcements encouraging and maintaining behavioral change at the individual level. For instance, Flynn et al. (1994) found that an intensive mass media campaign combined with a resistance skills school-based program was more effective than the school program alone in preventing cigarette smoking. A well-orchestrated, intensive mass media campaign was mounted to reach the target audience of young adolescents. Up to 450 paid television and radio advertisements were broadcast each year to saturate the media with antismoking messages.

The Midwestern Prevention Program (MPP) developed by Pentz and colleagues (Johnson et al., 1990) is one widely cited model for community intervention. MPP begins with a school-based resistance skills program offered during the sixth grade. MPP also includes four other major components that are phased in over the 5-year course of the intervention and involves families, peers, schools, and the general community. For instance, there are components promoting use of peer leaders, parent involvement, community organization, and a mass media campaign. Parents first become involved by helping their children complete school homework assignments related to drugs, and parents also receive training in drug prevention activities and communication skills. Schools seek to develop and enforce more effective antidrug policies and various community groups and members work with parents and students in the other aspects of MPP.

The importance of a communitywide intervention is nicely illustrated in findings from the Class of 1989 Study (Klepp, Kelder, & Perry, 1995; Perry et al., 1992). The Class of 1989 Study was part of a larger communitywide health promotion program, the Minnesota Heart Health Program (MHHP). MHHP consisted of various community-based activities to change behavior in three main areas: eating habits, physical activity levels, and smoking. Many health agencies and community groups participated and the local media cooperated in advertising and supporting different activities. The Class of 1989 Study was a school-based program directed at changing children's behavior in the same three areas targeted by MHHP, as well as two additional behaviors: alcohol and marijuana use. Since the latter two drugs were not targeted in the larger MHHP intervention, the investigators had a chance to compare the short- and long-term effects of a school-only versus a school-plus-community intervention for the same cohort of students.

Overall, positive results were obtained for all five areas targeted in the school program immediately following completion of the intervention (Klepp et al., 1995). These positive results were maintained at follow-up, but only in those areas covered by the communitywide intervention: eating habits, physical activity, and smoking (Kelder, Perry, Lytle, & Klepp, 1995; Perry et al., 1992). In other words, the immediate reduction in alcohol and marijuana use demonstrated by the Class of 1989 Study participants was not sustained over time. The lesson from the Class of 1989 Study seems clear: The absence of environmental factors that reinforce and support individual changes in behavior makes long-term change difficult to achieve.

Project Northland was another effort that combined a school-based and communitywide intervention (Perry et al., 1996). Project Northland attempted to change individual behaviors and the social environment simultaneously to discourage alcohol use and promote social norms about not using alcohol. Behavioral curricula presented by peers and teachers were used in the school to teach students how to resist social pressures to drink and how to intervene in their community to reduce alcohol use. Students and parents participated in home activities by following program manuals that encouraged parent–child discussions of alcohol use and its consequences. Teens and adult volunteers organized alcohol-free activities in the community. Finally, a communitywide task force was formed to coordinate the activities of local groups to be a positive influence on teen drinking. The task force was successful in its efforts to pass local ordinances regarding sales of alcohol to minors and met with local merchants about their sale practices. Other local businesses were involved and offered discounts to students who pledged to be alcohol-free.

At the end of the 3-year intervention, 19% fewer program than control students reported any drinking at all within the past month. The intervention was twice as effective for students who had never drunk alcohol than among those who had tried alcohol before the program began. One important effect occurred that signaled a major change in perceptions of peer alcohol use. Compared to controls, program students were significantly more likely to believe that many of their peers drank at the beginning of the intervention, and they were significantly less likely to hold the same belief at the end of intervention. This finding may signal a central mechanism through which program effects might be mediated: perceived social norms about peer drinking.

Another intervention combining school and community components that has achieved impressive long-term effects is the North Karelia Youth Project (NKYP) (Vartiainen et al., 1990). NKYP occurred in Finland and began as a communitywide intervention for the general population. It focused on reducing cardiovascular risk through a variety of screening, educational, mass media, and health-focused programs. Reducing smoking and improving diet were emphasized. After this community program had been in existence for 5-years, a school-based component, NKYP, was added specifically to prevent smoking in 13- to 15-year-olds, and long-term follow-up has concentrated on the impact of this school-based smoking program.

NKYP was a resistance skills training program begun in seventh grade and conducted over two successive school years by peer leaders, project staff, or teachers, depending on the school district and its resources. Figure 4.1 presents the impressive outcome data collected over successive follow-up periods on students who were nonsmokers at the

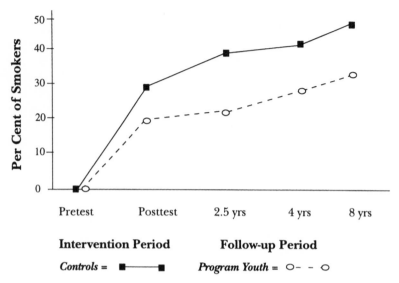

Figure 4.1.   Percentage of program and control youth in the North Karelia Project reporting any amount of smoking. Data are from Vartiainen et al. (1990) and are based on nonsmokers at the beginning of the intervention.

beginning of the intervention (Vartiainen et al., 1990). The program was successful at reducing the percentage of new smokers at all time points. In fact, 8 years after the intervention ended, rates of smoking were still 28% lower among program than nonprogram youth (34% vs. 47%, respectively). The 8-year follow-up is particularly important. The odds are only one in eight that someone over the age of 18 will become a regular smoker (Elders et al., 1994). Since the last NKYP follow-up data were collected when the sample participants were between 21 to 23 years old, program effects have extended beyond the critical high-risk period for smoking.

Finally, one study presented in Table 4.1 is a good example of how community interventions can be tailored for specific cultural groups, in this case, American Plains Indians (Cheadle et al., 1995). Several risk factors characterized the tribe of Native Americans targeted for intervention including an unemployment rate close to 70%, a suicide rate that was more than 20 times the national rate, a high percentage of single-parent families (56%), and low levels of parental education. A 5-year communitywide program was primarily directed at reducing alcohol use and abuse but also included other drugs. There were 14 major components to this multifaceted intervention directed at youth, parents, and the entire community such as education and skill-building programs for parents and children of all ages offered in both school and community settings, youth leadership and summer employment programs, special community fairs and events, and public campaigns regarding drug use. An important feature of this program was the use of tribal elders to plan and administer many program activities in ways that suited the norms and values of the Native-American population. Although results did not always reach customary levels of significance due to low statistical power, several major changes were noted following intervention. Compared to controls, program adolescents reported almost twice as much reduction in binge drinking, they were less likely to begin drinking before the 9th grade, and they were less likely to be a passenger in a car driven by someone who had been drinking. With respect to other drugs, program youth showed less use of marijuana and smokeless tobacco.

Three important issues need clarification in future drug prevention programs: (1) determining the best timing and duration for interventions; (2) assessing whether program effects generalize across populations and settings; and (3) identifying what elements contribute to short- and long-term impact. Each of these issues is now briefly discussed.

Timing and Duration

Both the timing and duration of intervention are important. Most interventions begin when students are in grades 5–8, since this is the time when many youth begin experimenting with drugs. Early intervention is important. The earlier that drug taking occurs, the greater the risk for subsequent use (Hawkins et al., 1992). Some data indicate that the most durable results are obtained among program youth who were not taking drugs when the intervention began (Vartiainen et al., 1990).

Brief interventions rarely achieve positive effects, especially over the long term. All of the programs in Table 4.1 lasted several years. Typically, a program is begun one year and booster sessions or additional components are offered in subsequent school years. Stretching the intervention over several years makes sense from a developmental standpoint. As children enter adolescence, there are several factors they must contend with such as puberty, development of opposite-sex relationships, increased pressure from peers coupled with a need for peer acceptance, and a desire to become more independent from parents. Therefore, a continuing intervention can incorporate these developmental factors into the program over time, and thus be more attuned to the immediate needs of youth. Therefore, a general recommendation is to begin the intervention early (before youth have started experimenting with drugs) and continue the program in some fashion over subsequent years.

Program Generalization

Investigators are beginning to document that the better programs do have wide applicability. For instance, researchers have demonstrated that: (1) program training manuals can be developed so that local staff can implement interventions effectively with limited consultation; (2) teachers, college students, local community volunteers, and peers can be used as change agents; (3) programs can be offered at various grade levels ranging from elementary through high school; (4) students in rural, suburban, and urban areas benefit from intervention; (5) many schools and sometimes entire school districts from different states can use a program successfully; and (6) specific programs can be effectively modified to suit the needs and lifestyles of different cultural and ethnic groups.

Effective Program Elements

All successful contemporary programs are multidimensional interventions, making it impossible to identify which components produce which outcomes. For instance, in addition to the program components already mentioned such as skills training, many programs present accurate information about drugs in such a way as to counteract misconceptions or misperceptions about peer drug use. This is done because youth frequently have the erroneous belief that most of their peers use drugs, and thus that drug use is acceptable and will be supported or reinforced. Programs also provide social support for not using drugs, involve parents in different ways, ask students to make public commitments not to use drugs, reinforce behavior change, and modify local social norms and policies about drugs. Future investigators must clarify how different program elements contribute to outcome.

A Special Word about Smoking

Programs to prevent cigarette smoking are valuable as both drug and physical health interventions. There is a general progression in drug taking as many youth first experiment with alcohol and cigarettes before moving on to other types of drugs (cocaine, marijuana, and so on). Therefore, cigarettes and alcohol are often identified as *gateway drugs* and are targeted in drug programs. Not all children who try alcohol or cigarettes move on to other drugs, of course, but reducing drinking and smoking can lessen the likelihood of future use of other drugs.

Cigarette smoking also has several health consequences because it is associated with increased mortality and morbidity in connection with lung cancer, coronary heart disease, stroke, and various respiratory diseases. Approximately 3000 teenagers start smoking each day in the United States, and eventually one out of every four of them will die from a smoking-related disease (United States Department of Health and Human Services, 1990). Therefore, smoking prevention programs can have a strong impact on the physical health status of a large segment of the population. Chapter 5 discusses smoking cessation programs for pregnant women and efforts to reduce young children's exposure to secondhand smoke.

Drug Use versus Misuse

It is important to distinguish use from the misuse or risky use of drugs. Although even limited use of some drugs such as tobacco, cocaine, or inhalants can endanger physical or psychological health, this is not the case with alcohol. Light or moderate drinking has not been associated with any serious health risks. It is true that if youth never drink, they will never experience any problems associated with alcohol use; but it is unrealistic to expect drug interventions to eliminate alcohol use entirely. Therefore, program evaluations should include data on how changes in drug use are associated with sexual behavior, driving, or school performance. Some studies are now beginning to report positive program effects in these areas (Cheadle et al., 1995; Hansen & Graham, 1991).

Gap between Research and Practice

Schools are the most common site for drug prevention and most schools offer some type of program. Unfortunately, many school programs are short, didactic offerings that have never been systematically evaluated and are probably of dubious impact. The most widely used school-based program is Project DARE, which has been used in more than 50% of all school districts. Project DARE has become very popular in large part because the program is federally funded and conducted by police officers. It does not cost the schools anything to host this program.

Unfortunately, evaluations of Project DARE indicate that this program does not significantly change student drug use (Ennett, Tobler, Ringwalt, & Flewelling, 1994).

It is a challenge to convince some schools of the need for extensive and intensive interventions to prevent drug use. Many districts have become comfortable with very brief programs that satisfy educational mandates requiring that some form of drug prevention program be in place. National campaigns that propose simple but ineffectual solutions (e.g., "Just Say No to Drugs") compound the problem. Fortunately, as this chapter indicates, several researchers have been successful in encouraging schools to adopt and support more sophisticated and successful interventions.

SUMMARY

There has been substantial improvement over the past 25 years in the theory and corresponding execution of drug prevention programs concomitant with an increase in the number of programs that report success in changing drug-related behaviors. Early unsuccessful programs based on the assumption that imparting information about drugs would change attitudes and behaviors have given way to more sophisticated psychosocial interventions that target multiple social influences on drug use. As a result, initial pessimism over the impact of drug prevention programs that followed the first round or two of interventions in the 1960s has now been replaced by guarded optimism that success is possible.

There have been several convincing examples that the number of youth who use drugs and the quantity of drugs consumed can be substantially reduced and that programs can have lasting effects. Most effective programs have been multidimensional interventions that make it impossible to determine exactly why a program is successful. Effective programs often emphasize two major themes. First, systematic skill training is used to help youth make careful decisions and resist social pressures to take drugs and perhaps to change their perceptions of the acceptability and normative use of drugs. Second, social and environmental factors influence drug use. Modeling by peers and adults, social norms, and active participation in community antidrug programs seem to contribute to long-term changes in drug-related behavior. Legislation and taxation as methods to reduce access to drugs are other approaches that have value (see Chapter 9).

5

Programs to Improve Physical Health

INTRODUCTION

Various data summarized by the Children's Defense Fund (1995) present a dramatic snapshot of the health of America's children and suggest what improvements can be made. For example, the infant mortality rate in the United States lags behind 21 other industrialized countries. The incidence of low birth weight, which places infants at heightened risk for death and long-term disability, was actually higher in 1992 (7.1% of all births) than it was in 1980 (6.8%). Nearly one out of every four pregnant mothers does not obtain early prenatal care, thus exposing themselves and their infants to increased risk of death and disease. Only two thirds of America's young children are fully immunized against preventable childhood diseases, meaning that there are millions of youngsters unnecessarily exposed to such diseases as measles, tetanus, polio, and hepatitis B. Approximately 22% of all children live in substandard housing that may not provide suitable sleeping facilities, adequate warmth, or physical safety. In addition, there are an estimated 1 million homeless and runaway children whose basic needs for physical safety, food, and shelter are inconsistently met.

Poverty is one variable consistently related to health status, and 1993 figures indicated that 27% of children under the age of 3, or approximately 15.7 million children, lived in poverty. Compared to other children, children from low-income households are twice as likely to die from birth defects, are at least two times more likely to have growth and developmental problems and severe physical and mental disabilities, and are five to six times more likely to die from diseases during infancy and childhood. There are approximately three times more black and Latino than white children who live in poverty. Poor children are concentrated in single-parent households, and 54% of children in single-mother households live in poverty.

Promoting physical health is important because a child's health status has consequences for all aspects of child development. Poor physical health places children at risk for numerous social, psychological, and academic problems and creates stress and burden for family caregivers (Lavigne & Faier-Routman, 1992). In summary, much can be done to improve the health of children, and those from low-income and single-parent households are especially at risk.

This chapter focuses on physical health and is developmentally arranged. Programs for infants and young children, for elementary school-age children, and, finally, for adolescents are discussed in succession. There is some overlap between programs for the latter two age groups, but the last section concentrates on sex education and efforts to prevent adolescent pregnancy and AIDS.

PROGRAMS FOR PREGNANT WOMEN AND YOUNG CHILDREN

Smoking during Pregnancy

One factor clearly related to both maternal and infant health is smoking. Smoking during pregnancy increases the risk of low birth weight, spontaneous abortions, premature delivery, and various medical complications during pregnancy. Almost one in five women (18%) continues to smoke during pregnancy, despite the risks to themselves and their offspring (Floyd, Rimer, Giovino, Mullen, & Sullivan, 1993). Because of the extent and danger of smoking during pregnancy, Floyd et al. (1993) concluded that "Prenatal smoking cessation could make significant contributions to the improvement of maternal and infant health and could save the health-care system millions of dollars" (p. 381).

The Floyd et al. (1993) review of prenatal smoking cessation programs conducted in the United States, Canada, Great Britain, and Sweden indicated that the majority of programs (10 of 13) were successful, although there was considerable variation in outcomes. Smoking quit rates for pregnant women have ranged from 3 to 32%. The more effective programs have been carefully implemented, multisession programs that emphasize behavioral change strategies. Clients learn how to apply self-monitoring, self-reinforcement, and stimulus control procedures by such practices as counting each cigarette smoked, setting realistic goals that slowly reduce the number of cigarettes consumed over time, smoking only in specific locations, and rewarding themselves for reaching personal goals. There is clearly room for improvement in interventions, since at best only one third of smokers have quit during pregnancy. Nevertheless, even modest reductions in the number of pregnant women who smoke can improve health and can be cost-effective, yielding over $45.00 in benefits for every dollar in program costs (see Chapter 8 for details).

Two well-done, randomized clinical trials illustrate the applicability of smoking cessation programs within public health clinics and health maintenance organizations. Windsor et al. (1993) evaluated the impact of a brief behavioral intervention conducted at four public health maternity clinics serving mostly low-income African-American women. During brief personal contacts, a nurse counselor emphasized the importance of not smoking during pregnancy, taught the mothers how to apply self-control strategies, and provided each mother with a self-help manual. Follow-up letters were also sent containing testimonials and strategies used by mothers who successfully quit, and a buddy system was available to provide social support for smoking cessation efforts. Significantly more experimental than control mothers quit smoking (14.3% vs. 8.5%, respectively).

The second randomized study was conducted in a health maintenance organization serving families of diverse socioeconomic status and ethnicity (Ershoff, Quinn, Mullen, & Lairson, 1990). This intervention also combined behaviorally oriented self-help materials and personal contacts conducted by a health educator. Almost three times more experimental than control women quit smoking by the end of their pregnancy (22.2% vs. 8.6%, respectively). Most importantly, there were 42% fewer low birth weight infants born to experimental mothers.

Passive Smoking Programs

It is also important to intervene after the birth of a child, because of the detrimental health effects of passive smoking (exposure to tobacco smoke in the air that is breathed, which is also sometimes called involuntary smoking or secondhand smoke). Passive smoking is believed to be responsible for between 150,000 to 300,00 cases of lower respiratory tract infections in young children, requiring up to 15,000 hospitalizations each year. Passive smoking exacerbates asthmatic conditions, reduces lung growth in young children, and may also affect cardiovascular health and increase later risk for various cancers. Passive smoking can also indirectly affect children's academic functioning by increasing school absenteeism rates by up to 40%. Furthermore, many children are at risk. More than half of all children under five in the United States are exposed in some way to passive smoking (Samet, Lewit, & Warner, 1994).

One large-scale study involving 128 pediatricians from 49 different private pediatric services found that it was possible to incorporate a smoking cessation program into well-baby clinic visits (Wall, Severson, Andrews, Lichtenstein, & Zoref, 1995). Pediatricians advised mothers about the effects of passive smoking and distributed self-help materials either at a single visit or during the course of four different well-baby checkups. A 6-month follow-up indicated that the lengthier intervention was more than twice as successful in getting mothers to stop smoking and was also more effective in preventing relapse among those who had stopped smoking during pregnancy.

In another investigation, nurses conducted four 45-minute home visits to educate new mothers about the dangers of passive smoke and to teach them methods to reduce their newborn's exposure to tobacco smoke (Greenberg et al., 1994). Information on smoking cessation programs available in the local community was provided to mothers who wished such information, but the intervention did not insist that the mother had to stop smoking. For example, smoking mothers were advised to not smoke in the infant's presence, to move the infant away from any sources of smoke, to ask people not to smoke in the same room or same car as the infant, and to sit in nonsmoking sections whenever possible. The home visits occurred during the child's first 6 months of life. A 6-month follow-up found that children of smoking mothers were exposed to 38% less tobacco smoke and experienced 42% fewer persistent lower respiratory symptoms than controls.

Although the preceding programs focusing on mothers' behaviors obtained some success, environmental interventions also are needed to reduce the risks of passive smoking in all settings with children. Current community education and mass media campaigns regarding smoking usually fail to highlight the detrimental effects of passive smoking on children. Chapter 9 discusses the impact of no-smoking laws and school policies regarding smoking, but here it is important to note that environments such as child day care centers should not be ignored. For instance, only three states require licensed day care centers to be smoke-free indoors; only a little over half of all centers (55%) are smoke free both indoors and outdoors (Samet et al., 1994).

Other Interventions for Families with Young Children

Table 5.1 presents some details on three exemplary health interventions for mothers of young children. These programs were chosen to represent home-visiting programs, a combination of home- and community-based services, and a clinic-based program. Each is now briefly described.

Home Visiting

The home-visiting program conducted in Elmira, New York, has become a widely cited intervention because of its careful design, execution, and evaluation and its ability to produce a broad array of positive health outcomes (Olds & Kitzman, 1993). Basically, this program provided health, parenting, and social support services by sending visitors into families' homes. The Elmira study sample contained a large number of white, first-time mothers, many of whom were under 19 years of age, single parents, and of low-income status.

**Table 5.1. Representative Health Programs
for Pregnant Women and Young Children**

Program	Target group	Intervention/main components	Major outcomes
Olds & Kitzman (1993)[a]	Young, single, low-income mothers	Home visiting to help infant and mother; health care, parent training, social support	Mothers received more prenatal services, returned to school and worked more frequently; children displayed better cognitive functioning
Infant Health and Development Program (1990)	Mothers with low-birth-weight premature infants	Home visiting and community services to help infant and mother; health care, parent training, and child preschool program	Children displayed better cognitive functioning and fewer behavioral problems; mothers more frequently working
O'Sullivan and Jacobsen (1992)	Young, single, low-income mothers	Clinic-based counseling for mothers	Mothers attended more well-baby checkups, children more fully immunized

[a]This intervention also reduced rates of child maltreatment. See Chapter 7.

Two home-visiting interventions that began during the 30th week of the mother's pregnancy and varied in intensity and duration were evaluated along with an untreated control group. In the first treatment condition, mothers were visited during their pregnancy, whereas in the second treatment group mothers received continuing visits until the child was 2 years of age. The home visits had two primary goals: (1) to promote mothers' ability to understand and respond to their children's health and social needs, and (2) to increase the social support received by the mother. In the latter case, home visitors provided direct support to mothers and helped them secure additional support from friends, relatives, and neighbors.

In general, the more intensive 2-year home-visiting condition was more effective, and in most cases, positive findings were still in evidence for both children and mothers at a 2-year follow-up, that is, when the children were about 4 years old. During pregnancy, mothers in the experimental group made greater use of available prenatal health services and attended more childbirth education classes. At the end of pregnancy, experimental mothers smoked fewer cigarettes, had better nutrition, and experienced fewer obstetrical complications such as kidney infections. Not one mother in the youngest experimental age group (14–16 years old) gave birth to a low birth weight infant (i.e., < 2500 grams), whereas 11.76% of the youngest controls did. At the end of pregnancy, experimental mothers also reported receiving more social support from partners and friends.

At the end of the 2-year intervention, home observations indicated that experimental mothers provided more effective play materials and better cognitive and language stimulation to their children; psychological evaluations indicated that their children had IQ scores 9 points higher than the controls. (There were also positive outcomes relative to child maltreatment and child injuries that favored the experimental group; these are described in Chapter 7.)

There were also positive changes in the mothers' lives. At the 2-year follow-up, the experimental mothers without a high school diploma had returned to school more quickly than control mothers. Poor, unmarried mothers had worked 82% more months during their child's first 4 years of life, spent 40% fewer days on welfare, had 43% fewer subsequent pregnancies, and had delayed the onset of a later pregnancy by an average of 1 year.

Home and Community-Based Services

The Infant Health and Development Program (IHDP) is a large-scale, ongoing investigation devoted to preventing developmental and health problems in low birth weight (< 2500 grams) premature infants (Infant Health and Development Program, 1990). As of October 1994, almost 1000 children ($n = 985$) drawn from eight collaborating sites throughout the United States have been studied from birth up through age 5. The 3-year intervention combines an early community-based childhood development program, family training and support services that are offered through home visiting, and follow-up medical care. IHDP begins when the infant is discharged from the neonatal nursery. Home visiting occurs weekly during the child's first year and biweekly for the next 2 years. The child attends a 5-day a week early childhood cognitive stimulation program between the ages of 1 and 3, and at the same time weekly parent groups are conducted. The parent groups provide social support and guidance in child rearing, address health and safety concerns, and deal with families' individual concerns and needs.

Evaluations of IHDP indicate the importance of addressing participant characteristics and conducting follow-up of program effects. The IHDP protocol created two subgroups of low birth weight infants, a heavier weight group (between 2000 and 2500 grams in weight), and a lighter group (< 2000 grams). Immediately after the conclusion of the 3-year intervention, significant effects for both weight groups compared to the controls appeared on IQ tests, with effects twice as large for the heavier than for the lighter birth weight group (13.2 vs. 6.6 IQ points, respectively). At 2-year follow-up, however, only the heavier weight group had maintained its significant IQ difference over corresponding controls.

Immediately following the intervention, mothers in both weight categories reported their children had significantly fewer behavior problems than controls. At this point, 26% fewer experimental than control children in both weight categories had behavior problems in the clinically significant range, but 2 years later there were no significant behavioral between-group differences between experimental and control children for either weight group (Brooks-Gunn et al., 1994).

Family variables also influenced outcomes. Families with the highest levels of program participation were almost seven times less likely than those who participated the least to have a child whose intellectual functioning fell into the range of mental retardation (Ramey et al., 1992). Children whose mothers had a high school education or less benefited the most (Brooks-Gunn, Gross, Kraemer, Spiker, & Shapiro, 1992).

Finally, positive effects were also noted for mothers. Although there were no significant effects in enhancing mothers' level of education or reducing the percentage of those receiving public assistance, mothers in IHDP did work significantly longer than controls (Brooks-Gunn, McCormick, Shapiro, Benasich, & Black, 1994). This effect was strongest for mothers with a high school education or less, which may be particularly important, since mothers with less formal schooling probably have the most difficult time finding suitable employment.

The IHDP program illustrates how critical it is to assess outcomes in relation to characteristics of program participants. Unless the target population is homogeneous, it is likely that the intervention will affect participants differently and these differences need to be understood. In the case of IHDP, it appears that both characteristics of the child and mother are important. Identifying which participants derive the most and the least benefits from an intervention is important in deciding how to improve the program or to disseminate it into other settings. It will be interesting to see how the results for IHDP unfold over time as the experimental and control cohorts progress through the elementary school years.

Clinic-Based Services

The third study listed in Table 5.1 is an example of a successful clinic-based program (O'Sullivan & Jacobsen, 1992). A special attempt was made to convince young, unmarried African-American adolescent mothers of the need for routine medical care for their infant as well as the necessity of continuing in school and delaying future childbearing. A multidisciplinary team of social workers, nurses, and pediatricians counseled the young mothers on effective family planning methods and appropriate infant care practices during routine well-baby checkups. Phone calls and letters were also sent to all mothers in the experimental group to prompt the mothers to reschedule any missed appointments.

The intervention did not improve the proportion of mothers who returned to school by 18 months after the birth of their first child, but several other significant effects were observed. Compared to controls, experimental mothers were twice as likely to have attended well baby checkups, twice as likely to have their child fully immunized, and were half as likely to have had a repeat pregnancy.

Guidelines for Effective Early Health Intervention

The programs discussed in the previous section are only a few among the hundreds that have been conducted in medicine, education, and public health to improve the health status of young children and families. Such programs have been called maternal and infant health programs, early intervention and early childhood education, family support programs, and home-visiting programs. Although these interventions have originated in different disciplines and have different titles, they often overlap in terms of their general philosophy or orientation, which types of health-related services are offered, and what populations are served.

The following discussion attempts to integrate the perspectives offered by several authors (Chamberlin, 1988; Dunst, Trivette, & Thompson, 1991; Olds & Kitzman, 1993) with my own analysis of the relevant literatures in order to offer three guidelines for increasing the success of health interventions for families with young children. Table 5.2 presents details on these guidelines. This material is presented as a guide for effective action rather than definitive research conclusions. Results have varied across programs, outcomes, and participants, and more work is needed to tease out the potent factors operating in effective interventions. Furthermore, some programs will vary in order to achieve specific goals. Nevertheless, results from the most successful programs have converged to suggest that certain principles should be given prominent consideration.

Guideline 1: Target High-Risk Groups

High-risk groups seem to profit the most from intervention. In general, the risk groups most in need are low-income families. These families often have the following additional characteristics: a single-parent household, young maternal age, low level of maternal education, minority status, and residence in an impoverished inner-city neighborhood or rural setting. Some investigators have specifically targeted first-time mothers in low-income households for intervention. Because programs need to be intense and of relatively long duration (see guideline 3 below), selecting high-risk groups for intervention is usually preferable to offering an universal intervention for the whole community. Few communities have the resources to treat everyone.

Guideline 2: Consider Health in Broad Terms

Successful interventions usually adopt a broad view of health that encompasses physical, social, and cognitive dimensions and the major focus tends to change over time in line with the child and family's development. For instance, during pregnancy there is a primary focus on physical health to prevent serious obstetric and birth complications. Early prenatal care, proper maternal nutrition, and eliminations of unhealthy maternal habits (e.g., smoking and drinking) are typically emphasized. Following the birth of the child, the focus often shifts to

Table 5.2. Guidelines for Effective Health Programs
for Families with Young Children

Guideline 1. Target high-risk populations: Those at higher risk for various child and family
. negative outcomes seem to profit the most from intervention.
I. Major risk factors:
    A. Poverty
    B. Young maternal age
    C. Single-parent status
    D. Family factors: e.g., highly stressed families, parents with poor child-rearing
        skills, drug problems, depression, or other pathology
    E. Residence in an impoverished neighborhood

Guideline 2. Develop a broad orientation toward health and help the entire family: View
health as a combination of physical, social, psychological, and cognitive dimensions.
Provide comprehensive services to achieve multiple overlapping goals. Develop
services for caregivers as well as children. The entire family requires assistance.
I. Possible child-focused services
    A. Major targets before birth: Prevent low birth weight, prematurity, obstetric and
        birth complications by helping pregnant mother:
        1. Receive early prenatal health care
        2. Improve nutrition
        3. Eliminate unhealthy behaviors (e.g., smoking, drinking, unsafe sexual
            practices)
    B. Multiple targets after birth:
        1. Physical health: Prevent childhood illnesses
            a. Well-baby checkups
            b. Proper immunizations
        2. Promote social and cognitive development:
            a. Train mothers in infant stimulation activities
            b. As child develops, promote child-rearing skills
            c. Offer a preschool program to promote school readiness
        3. Injury prevention
            a. Train parents in home safety
II. Possible adult-focused services
    A. Family planning services to delay subsequent pregnancies
    B. Vocational or job training
    C. Promote educational achievement
    D. Provide social support: Social support can reduce the stress of parenting and help
        adults deal with other personal, social, or economic stresses.

Guideline 3. Emphasize effective service delivery practices: It makes a difference when
and where services are offered, by whom, and for how long:
A. Begin during pregnancy or immediately after birth
B. Think in terms of years rather than weeks of intervention
C. Use well-training and supervised change agents
D. Consider providing at least some home-based services

teaching the new parent proper infant care practices and emphasizing the importance of well-baby checkups, meeting immunization schedules, and principles of home safety to reduce the risk of unintentional injury. Parents also learn how to respond to and stimulate infant behaviors in order to foster a secure infant–mother attachment bond, which can form the basis for a good parent–child relationship. As the child grows, parents are taught effective child-rearing skills to handle everyday management problems and prevent serious behavioral difficulties, and parents also learn how to stimulate their child's social and cognitive development to promote their child's school readiness. In some cases, the child is also enrolled in a preschool program to prepare the child for school entry.

Successful programs also provide adult- as well as child-focused services. The needs of parents as adults are attended to by providing social support and family planning services and discussing vocational and educational plans. Many programs are guided by the view that the child profits when the family system is enhanced or strengthened; thus adult caregivers need to become confident and skillful advocates for themselves and their offspring. In summary, a multidimensional intervention that addresses the physical, social, cognitive, and personal needs of all family members is needed.

Guideline 3: Emphasize Effective Service Delivery Practices

It makes a difference when and where services are offered, by whom, and for how long. For instance, earlier and lengthier interventions are generally more successful. Many effective programs begin during pregnancy or immediately after birth and maintain contact with families for several years. The intensity of intervention is high initially and diminishes over time. For instance, multiple weekly phone and personal contacts are usually provided initially, and these are gradually modified to once a week, biweekly, and monthly arrangements.

Service providers must be well trained. Paraprofessionals recruited from the local community have been used successfully, but many programs have relied on pediatricians, nurses, or certified early childhood educators to conduct the bulk of the program.

Finally, providing at least some services through a home-visiting program should be considered, although this does not mean that clinic-based programs are never effective (e.g., O'Sullivan & Jacobsen, 1992). Nevertheless, there are two important advantages to home visiting. First, more of the target population can be reached because the intervention in brought into recipients' homes. This overcomes many of the barriers or difficulties involved in accessing services, particularly for low-income families. For instance, one study of low-income pregnant teenagers found that compared to clinic-based services, home visiting reached a higher percentage of high-risk adolescents and promoted a higher level of prenatal care (Julnes, Konefal, Pindur, & Kim, 1994). Second, the components of home visiting can be tailored to suit each family. As the home visitor gains an appreciation for each unique home situation, different services can be emphasized at different times in accordance with the family's needs.

PROGRAMS FOR SCHOOL-AGE CHILDREN

The need for health programs continues as children develop. Up to 30% of school-age children have elevated cholesterol levels, 5% have hypertension, up to 30% are obese, up to 60% of youth do not get adequate exercise, and approximately 20% of high school seniors are regular smokers. The nutritional intake of many children is too high in fat and sodium and too low in recommended vitamins and minerals. One striking statistic is that by age 12, an estimated 60% of all children have at least one risk factor for coronary heart disease (see Cheung & Richmond, 1995; Resnicow et al., 1992). Therefore, some important targets for health interventions are to improve nutritional intake and exercise levels and to prevent youth from smoking.

The exact criteria that should be used to determine positive physical health and the long-term effect of childhood programs on adult health status have to be clarified. However, many authors have stressed the importance of childhood interventions because of the difficulty in changing adults' unhealthy behaviors. Enduring changes in adult habits related to smoking, drinking, eating, and exercise levels are difficult to achieve (Kaplan, 1984). Therefore, it makes sense to intervene early when children's attitudes and understanding of health and prevention are developing in order to help them initiate what may become lifelong patterns of healthy behaviors.

Transformation of School-Based Health Education

Schools have incorporated some form of health education into their curricula as far back as the early 1900s when children were taught basic information about hygiene and communicable diseases. For many years, most health education rested on the belief that the imparting of information would change behavior; but as with other areas of prevention, this assumption was found wanting. Simply informing people of how to prevent disease and improve their health rarely leads to significant behavior change. In contrast, contemporary theory and practice in health education emphasizes action-oriented interventions to change health-related practices. Most successful programs have emphasized one or both of the following two important principles: (1) children need to be carefully trained and reinforced if they are to develop and maintain new health-related behaviors (see Appendix A); and (2) intervention must move beyond classroom instruction to modify environmental factors that influence health practices. In the latter case, parent involvement, use of peers and the media, and various communitywide initiatives are incorporated into interventions.

Table 5.3 presents examples of successful health education programs for school-aged children, which are briefly described below. Generally, these programs can be divided according to those focusing on individual-level change through classroom training and those that also intervene to modify one or more aspects of the social environment.

A Landmark Study: SHEE

The School Health Education Evaluation (SHEE) was a landmark attempt at health education in elementary schools whose findings have strongly influenced the conduct of subsequent programs (Connell, Turner, & Mason, 1985). SHEE involved over 30,000 children from grades 4 to 7 drawn from over 1000 classrooms in 20 states. Four different health education programs that focused on reducing cardiovascular risk and promoting health were evaluated. Overall, the programs were twice as effective in modifying knowledge than behavior, but significant behavioral outcomes were obtained for two of the four programs. However, these overall results were not as important as additional data that identified three circumstances affecting program impact. First, students receiving 2 years of SHEE programs demonstrated significantly more behavioral gains than those who participated for only 1 year. Second, there were marked differences across participating sites in how well SHEE was implemented. Some teachers omitted critical portions of the programs. When the program was fully implemented, however, there were substantially more behavioral effects among participating students. Third, program intensity made a difference. The most stable and maximum program effects occurred after 50 hours of classroom instruction; moreover, significant effects for some programs did not begin to occur unless the program was offered for at least 20 hours and parents were involved, as the program model emphasized. In summary, SHEE

Table 5.3. Representative Health Programs for School-Age Children

Program	Target group	Intervention/main components	Major outcomes
Connell, Turner, & Mason (1985)	Grades 4–7	Four school-based health programs: diet and nutrition	Increased healthy behaviors, particularly among programs well implemented and over 20 hours in duration
Lombard et al. (1991)	Youth at public swimming pools	Modeling by lifeguards and goal-setting strategies	Fourfold increase in behaviors protecting against skin cancer
Kelder, Perry, & Klepp (1993)	Grades 6–10	School- and community-based program targeting nutrition, exercise and smoking	Improved exercise levels and nutrition; 39% fewer smokers
Perry et al. (1988)	Grade 3	School health program requiring parent involvement	Improved nutrition
Simons-Morton et al. (1988, 1991)	Grades 3 and 4	Classroom instruction coupled with changes in physical education and school cafeteria service	Increase in physical activity and improved nutrition
Writing Group for the DISC Collaborative Research Group (1995)	8 to 10 year olds	Community-based family counseling	Improved nutrition and lower cholesterol

outcome data clearly indicated that how well programs were conducted and for long can make an important difference. Brief or poorly implemented interventions are unlikely to be very effective. These lessons have been taken to heart by many subsequent health educators.

Protection against Skin Cancer

Because there is evidence of a causal link between excessive sun exposure and skin cancer, improving sun protection has become another topic for preventive health. Several sources describe the magnitude of the problem and possible solutions (Arthey & Clarke, 1995; Girgis, Sanson-Fisher, Tripodi, & Golding, 1993; Lombard, Neubauer, Canfield, & Winett, 1991).

In many parts of the world, the rate of skin cancer has doubled in the past 10 years and is at an alarming high level in Australia where two of three people are expected to develop at least one skin cancer in their lifetime. The most effective form of protection is to avoid ultraviolet radiation, that is, stay out of the sun. When this is impossible, however, the regular use of effective suncreeen (SPF $\geq$ 15) during the first two decades of life can reduce skin cancer risk by 78%. Sun protection is particularly important for younger people whose skin is more sensitive and who receive up to three times more ultraviolet radiation than adults.

Two studies, one based in the schools and the other in the community, illustrate successful approaches to increasing sun protection. In Australia, the effects of an educational intervention and a skill training intervention were compared (Girgis et al., 1993). The educational program consisted of a single didactic presentation on sun protection provided by an experienced cancer education staff member. Often this limited approach is used to deal with the problem of skin cancer. The more intensive 4-week skill training program incorporated active learning strategies to teach children about the risks of sun exposure and to help them problem solve potentially effective behavioral solutions. Children were also taught how to use a Solar Protection Behavior Diary to self-monitor their sun protection behaviors.

The didactic presentation had no significant behavioral effect. Once again, an exclusive informational approach did not change child behaviors. Students receiving the more intensive program, however, were more than twice as likely as those in the information condition to exercise a high level of solar protection immediately following the program and were three times more likely to do so at an 8-month follow-up.

Another study changed child and adolescent behavior over a

3-month period at two local public swimming pools by combining informational posters and prompting with modeling and daily feedback (Lombard et al., 1991). Informational flyers were first distributed to all pool patrons describing the risks of sun cancer and what can be done to protect oneself when at the pool. Following a brief training program, lifeguards modeled effective sun protection behaviors by wearing protective clothing, sitting under umbrellas, and using sunscreens. Daily feedback to all pool patrons was presented via posters displayed around the pool area. These feedback posters summarized what percentage of individuals on a previous day practiced the safe sun behaviors described on the flyers and asked those attending the pool on the present day to achieve a new and higher daily goal. Any child willing to sign a commitment card pledging they would practice the targeted behaviors was eligible to win T-shirts or hats at an upcoming raffle. Children and adolescents increased their use of two or more protective solar behaviors fourfold during the intervention.

The authors of both of the above studies in which an individual-level approach to behavioral change was used noted the potential of environmental interventions. For instance, Australian school policies permitting children to wear skirts and shorts increase exposure to the sun and could be changed. Lombard et al. (1991) noted that the construction of more shaded areas around swimming pools is a strategy that should be pursued to provide more people with protection against the sun.

Involving Parents: The Home Team

It makes sense that involving parents in health interventions would increase the impact and durability of program effects, because parents are in a position to be critical role models and reinforcing agents for children in terms of healthy practices and preventive behaviors. However, several investigators have encountered difficulty in involving parents in health interventions, particularly if they ask parents to attend meetings at school or the community. This is not surprising, since parents have reported that participating in such activities is not particularly attractive to them (Perry, Crockett, & Pirie, 1987).

Perry and colleagues have been one of the few groups that have successfully involved parents in health programs for their children. These researchers developed a home correspondence health program focusing on nutrition for young children, the Home Team (HT), which requires parents' participation (Crockett, Mullis, Perry, & Luepker, 1989). Children are rewarded at school as they complete health-related activities at home with their parents over a 5-week period. Parent participation rates of 77% or more have been achieved in HT studies, presumably because parents become motivated to help their children complete their schoolwork and earn desired incentives. HT has produced dual benefits in terms of significantly improving children's diets and changing parents' behaviors. After participating in HT, parents' attitudes toward the importance of diet improves, they talk more to their children about good eating habits, give their children more input into food choices, and have healthier foods on hand at home.

Class of 1989 Study Revisited

Before leaving the discussion of health programs for elementary children, findings for the Class of 1989 Study should be briefly reconsidered (Kelder, Perry, & Klepp, 1993). As the reader might recall, this study was originally described in Chapter 4 because it contained a school-based component focusing on alcohol and marijuana. In addition, the 5-year-long Class of 1989 Study targeted nutrition, physical exercise, and smoking, and this program was offered in the context of a larger communitywide intervention, which also emphasized the same three health issues. Students participating in the Class of 1989 Study did demonstrate both short- and long-term changes in levels of exercise, eating habits, and smoking rates. For instance, 2 years after the intervention ended, program students but not controls were exercising at a level recommended for cardiovascular fitness, that is, they were engaging in vigorous exercise at least three times a week (Kelder et al., 1993). Similarly, by the end of high school, program students had healthier eating habits than controls (Kelder et al., 1995) and 39% fewer students were smoking (Perry et al., 1992). Female students were more responsive to the intervention regarding exercise and nutrition than males. The developers of the Class of 1989 Study believed that the social norms, expectations, and reinforcements that were created in the local community were important contributors to the long-term changes observed in youths' healthy behaviors.

Organizational Change in Schools

The Go for Health Program (Simons-Morton, Parcel, Baranowski, Forthofer, & O'Mara, 1991; Simons-Morton, Parcel, & O'Mara, 1988) attempts to promote physical fitness and good nutrition in elementary schoolchildren. This program is innovative in integrating a classroom curriculum with organizational changes occurring in both the school food service and physical education program. The classroom instruction consists of six skill-training modules designed to teach third and fourth graders how to identify healthy from unhealthy foods and what types of physical activity will improve physical fitness. Children also learn how to self-monitor their levels of physical activity and food choices and they are reinforced for any positive changes they make in these areas.

The Go for Health team offers consultation to the food service and physical education department to achieve systemic changes in school practices. Members of the food service learn how to prepare more nutritious servings in the school cafeteria, and physical education teachers are helped to transform their classes to include more activities that improve physical fitness, such as aerobic exercises and dancing. The latter consultation is important because many physical education programs do not promote physical health through conditioning or exercise. Observations suggest that the average elementary student spends only 3½ minutes per class in moderate to vigorous physical activity (Simons-Morton, Taylor, Snider, & Huang, 1993).

Outcome studies indicate that Go for Health achieves its goals of promoting physical activity and better nutrition (Simons-Morton et al., 1988, 1991). Program children have demonstrated a fourfold increase in the time they spend in moderate to vigorous physical activity and they spend almost twice as much time in such activities as control students. Analyses of school lunches reflect reductions of 47%, 25%, and 13% in the intake of sodium, saturated, and total fat, respectively. Finally, a 1-year follow-up indicated that whereas the level of sodium intake increased over time by 18.5% in control schools, it decreased 31% in two experimental schools. Fat intake decreased only 5% in the former schools but 35% in Go for Health schools.

The Go for Health program illustrates how environmental interventions can be designed to complement change at the individual level. In the classroom children learn how to improve their physical and nutritional health, while the school environment is simultaneously being changed to reinforce and support children's new behaviors. Moreover, the organizational changes achieved in the school cafeteria and physical education department have the added benefit of affecting the entire school population year after year. Because of its environmental components, Go for Health has the potential to achieve more sustained changes in more schoolchildren than would be possible if the intervention was limited to classroom instruction for selected grade levels.

The nutritional value of many school lunch programs can certainly be improved. One survey of 545 public schools found that virtually none offered lunches that satisfied the guidelines of the United States Dietary Association (Children's Defense Fund, 1995). The food offered in many child care centers hardly fares better. Approximately 5 million children under the age of 6 eat meals at full- or part-time child care centers and the meals offered at these centers frequently fall short of recommended dietary allowances for young children (Briley, Roberts-Gray, & Rowe, 1993).

Child and Adolescent Trial for Cardiovascular Health

Findings from the Child and Adolescent Trial for Cardiovascular Health (CATCH) suggest that organizational changes in schools to improve health are possible on a wide scale (Luepker et al., 1996). CATCH was a randomized field trial involving over 5000 children from 96 schools in four states. The main program components were similar to the Simons-Morton et al. (1988, 1991) studies: a classroom component and organizational changes to improve the nutritional content of school lunches and the activities occurring in physical education classes. Some of the program schools also featured parent involvement similar to the Home Team intervention. CATCH began with third graders and continued for 3 years. The pattern of outcomes obtained from a variety of measures reflected program success. For instance, among the significant findings, the total fat content of school lunches fell by 18% in program schools but only 7% in control schools; dietary cholesterol levels fell by 8% among program students but rose 3% in controls. Compared to controls, program students reported significant improvements in their out-of-school eating patterns in terms of total and saturated fats and cholesterol intake. Both student reports and observations of physical education classes reflected significantly more vigorous physical activity occurring among program than among control students. Finally, CATCH was effective regardless of students' gender or ethnic group within the diverse study sample, suggesting that similar health interventions may be applicable in many different school systems.

Dietary Intervention Study in Children:
A Community-Based Intervention

In contrast to the other programs contained in Table 5.2 using a universal population approach (all children in the population are targeted), the Dietary Intervention Study in Children (DISC) is a community-based effort representing a high-risk (selective prevention) population approach (Writing Group for the DISC Collaborative Research

Group, 1995). DISC screened and selected for intervention only children at high risk for hypertension.

Families were recruited through private and public elementary schools, private pediatric practices, and health maintenance organizations. More than 44,000 8- to 10-year-old male and female children were screened at six collaborating sites throughout the United States, and those whose cholesterol levels were between the 80th and 98th percentiles adjusted for sex and age were targeted for intervention (n = 663). Children beyond the 98th percentile were not chosen because the investigators wanted to restrict their study to children for whom dietary managment of cholesterol (rather than medication) could be a recommended treatment.

Based on the child's initial eating patterns, DISC staff developed individualized dietary plans to be followed by the child and administered by the parents. The primary program consisted of a combination of 20 individual and group sessions occurring over a 1-year period in which a multidisciplinary staff (health educators, nutritionists, and behavior therapists) helped the children and parents keep to their dietary plans and goals. There were also a dozen booster or maintenance sessions conducted over the following two years and these sessions were further supplemented by periodic telephone contacts to answer questions and deal with specific problems.

At the end of the 3-year study, dietary total fat, saturated fat, and cholesterol levels decreased significantly in the intervention group compared to the controls. Equally impressive was the high level of family participation: Attendance averaged 90% or higher over the 3-year period. It is apparent that these investigators developed an intervention that was very acceptable to families.

SEX EDUCATION AND AIDS AND PREGNANCY PREVENTION

Programs for young people that address sexuality can be controversial. Although the majority of citizens favor sex education, some conservative and religious groups have been able to influence the type of education or research that is conducted on sexual topics. For example, from 1991 to 1995, over 400 local initiatives were mounted to limit the type of information that schools provide in sex education curricula (Ross & Kantor, 1995). Political pressures were influential in the decision made by the Secretary of Health and Human Services to cancel the American Teen Study, a research project funded by the National Institutes of Health that was about to investigate, among other health issues, adolescents' sexual behaviors (Gardner & Wilcox, 1993). Political factors were also instrumental in the drafting of the Adolescent and Family Act of 1981. This act only funds pregnancy prevention programs that have sexual abstinence as a primary goal, despite the absence of scientific data that such programs are effective for youth who are already sexually active. In summary, failure to understand and deal with potential opposition can lead to the undermining or blocking of programs containing sexual elements.

Nevertheless, sexual activity can be risky and may result in unwanted pregnancy, sexually transmitted diseases, or death through AIDS. It has been estimated that one in four sexually active teenagers contracts a sexually transmitted disease each year (Alan Guttmacher Institute, 1994); there are 1 million teenage pregnancies each year, and an adolescent pregnancy places both the mother and child at risk for a variety of long-term, negative social, educational, and health outcomes (Furstenberg, Brooks-Gunn, & Morgan, 1987). Because of the typically long incubation period between initial infection and the appearance of AIDS symptoms, the exact incidence of infection among adolescents is difficult to gauge. However, it appears that many adolescents are being infected (Henggeler, Melton, & Rodrigue, 1992). Therefore, it makes sense to design programs to prevent negative outcomes associated with sexual activity.

Characteristics of Effective Programs

Most systematic information on the impact of sexuality and pregnancy prevention programs has appeared within the past 10–15 years, and there is still much to be learned about how to influence young people's sexual behaviors. Nevertheless, there is some consensus among reviewers of sex education (Kirby et al., 1994), HIV/AIDS prevention (Kelly, 1995), and pregnancy prevention programs (Christopher, 1995) regarding the elements that seem to characterize successful programs:

1. There should be a focus on reducing risky sexual behaviors and increasing safe sexual practices. Basically, there are two ways to reduce risk: (1) not have sex, or (2) practice safe sex. For instance, if one is sexually active, safe practices that reduce the risk of AIDS would include using effective means of contraception during sexual intercourse, having sex with only one rather than multiple partners, and avoiding intercourse with intravenous drug users.
2. The timing of intervention must be consistent with program

goals. For instance, while sexual abstinence eliminates any risk from sexual behavior, it is often very difficult to convince youth who are already sexually active to cease their activity. Therefore, programs emphasizing abstinence have a better chance of success if they are begun before youth become sexually active (i.e., during the preteen years).

3. Youth must be trained systematically in skills related to safe sexual practices. Simply providing information will not change behavior. Social learning and cognitive behavioral techniques have been most successful in increasing sex-related skills. The most frequently targeted skills have included decision making, assertiveness, communication skills, and the correct use of contraception.

4. Multicomponent programs are needed. Adolescents frequently ignore or underestimate the risks associated with sexual behavior. Interventions that help youth integrate correct information and accurate perception of risk with the learning of new behaviors are more likely to achieve better results.

5. Environmental influences on sexual behavior should be stressed. In particular, positive family influences, peer behavior, and social or community norms emphasizing safe sexual practices should be enhanced.

6. Communitywide interventions that involve citizen coalitions, popular opinion leaders, the media, and so on may be necessary to sustain behavioral change over time.

7. Interventions must be tailored to suit the target population. Important variables to consider include gender, sexual orientation, minority group status, and religious values and background. It is unlikely that the same program will work equally well for all youth in all settings.

8. It is noteworthy that data indicate that preventive programs for young people do not increase rates of sexual activity, even if the program involves free distribution of condoms. This information may be helpful in countering the arguments of those who believe that teaching children about sex will increase sexual behavior.

Representative Programs

The studies summarized in Table 5.4 represent a range of successful interventions designed to modify sexual behaviors. These programs have varied in the specific groups targeted for intervention (e.g., junior high and high school students, adolescent runaways, pregnant mothers),

Table 5.4. Representative Programs in Sex Education and AIDS and Pregnancy Prevention

Study	Adolescent sample	Type of program	Major outcomes
Allen et al. (1994)	Junior and senior high school students from 66 schools	Classroom program and community activities	16% fewer course failures; 23% fewer suspensions; 41% fewer pregnancies
Rotheram-Borus et al. (1991)	Runaways staying in homeless shelter	Up to 20 small-group sessions	Greater use of condoms; less sexually risky behaviors overall
St. Lawrence et al. (1995)	African Americans recruited through public health clinic	Eight small-group sessions	Among virgins, one third as many began having sex; among nonvirgins, 36% more stopped sexual activity
Hobfoll et al. (1994)	Pregnant women from inner-city public health clinics	Four small-group sessions	Fewer risky and more safe sexual behaviors
Zabin et al. (1986)	Inner-city junior and senior high school students	School clinic offering counseling, sex ed, and health services	30% fewer pregnancies among program students vs. 58% more among controls

the setting for the program (e.g., schools, homeless shelters, and health clinics), and the level of intervention (individual and environmental programs are represented).

Sexuality and AIDS

A good demonstration of the relative benefits of skills training over an informational approach was provided by St. Lawrence and co-workers (1995). African-American adolescents were recruited through a local public health clinic to participate in one of two AIDS risk reduction programs: (1) an information-only condition that presented accurate information on AIDS and how to reduce risk, or (2) a program combining information with a skills-training approach in risk reduction. In the latter case, youth were systematically taught skills such as correct condom use, communication skills, and assertiveness in resisting unwanted sexual pressures. Youth also met with HIV-positive peers who discussed how their HIV status had affected their lives.

Only the skills-training approach changed youths' sexual behaviors, and both females and males profited. Role-playing assessments indicated that trained youth were more skillful in resisting coercive encounters and in insisting on safe sexual practices. Trained youth also reduced the frequency of unprotected intercourse, and 36% fewer teens were sexually active during the year following the program.

Another study targeted adolescent runaways who are at particularly high risk for AIDS because of their susceptibility to sexual victimization, prostitution, and drug use (Rotheram-Borus, Koopman, Haignere, & Davies, 1991). New admissions to New York City homeless shelters were recruited over a 2-year period and only 5% of potential participants refused. A 20-session skill-training program was conducted in the shelter and emphasized safe sexual practices. Trained youth demonstrated more consistent condom use and less frequent sexual activity; results were maintained over a 6-month follow-up period. As one might expect, shelters serve a transient population. Youth who attended more program sessions demonstrated greater change than those attending fewer sessions.

The study of pregnant women is listed in Table 5.4 to alert readers to the potential for AIDS prevention with this target group (Hobfoll, Jackson, Lavin, Britton, & Shepherd, 1994). Pregnant women who are HIV-positive can pass the infection on to the fetus; in 1993, 87% of the over 4700 children with AIDS were believed to have gotten the disease from their mother (Deren, Davis, Tortu, Beardsley, & Ahluwalia, 1995).

In the Hobfoll et al. (1994) study, single, pregnant women were recruited from three inner-city health clinics and participated in four 2-hour group sessions beginning during the women's second trimester of pregnancy. The intent of the program was to help women develop effective health care practices during pregnancy. Videotapes were used and served as a stimulus for group discussion and to model healthy behaviors. Social learning techniques were used to help women learn negotiation, communication, and assertiveness skills. Cognitive rehearsal strategies were also used to increase a sense of mastery and to heighten the perception of risk resulting from unhealthy practices. For instance, in this approach, women might be asked to imagine not using a condom during intercourse and later giving birth to a baby with the HIV virus.

Compared to controls, women participating in this program engaged in significantly fewer risky behaviors and practiced more safe sex behaviors (e.g., using condoms and discussing AIDS with their sexual partners). These differences were maintained at a 6-month follow-up, and the program was equally effective for African-American and Caucasian women. The Hobfoll et al. (1994) program is important in making several demonstrations: (1) pregnant women can be effectively recruited from community agencies to participate in AIDS prevention; (2) a brief, well-timed intervention can be effective; (3) results persist during the risk period of pregnancy and following the birth of the child; and (4) the program works equally well for at least two different populations (African Americans and Caucasians). The use of videotapes in this program also aides the standardized dissemination of this program into other settings.

Pregnancy Prevention

Two programs listed in Table 5.4 represent alternative strategies to reduce adolescent pregnancies. One program, Teen Outreach, has received national attention for its documented effectiveness in reducing teenage pregnancy. Teen Outreach is sponsored by the Association of Junior Leagues International and has been implemented in over 130 sites throughout the United States (Allen, Kuperminc, Philliber, & Herre, 1994; Philliber & Allen, 1992). Teen Outreach attempts to create viable life options for teens through a unique combination of community- and school-based components. In the former, adolescents spend time each week doing volunteer work of their choosing in one or more approved sites. This volunteer activity may involve work in hospital and nursing homes, tutoring younger students, or other types of community service. Having teens doing valuable volunteer work makes use of the helper therapy principle (Riessman, 1965), which maintains that people receive important benefits by helping others. The school-based component of Teen Outreach consists of a structured curriculum involving weekly discussions, exercises, and films devoted to critical developmental tasks of adolescence. Topics include understanding self and others, developing communication and problem-solving skills, and family stress and conflicts. Students enter the program at various times between grades 7 to 12. Trained teachers or guidance counselors function as facilitators and they coordinate students' school and community activities.

Teen Outreach has focused on preventing three major outcomes: school failure, school dropouts, and teen pregnancy. Data available on seven consecutive program cohorts indicate substantial reductions in these outcomes of between 15 and 50% (Philliber & Allen, 1992). For example, one recent evaluation comparing over 2000 program participants and nonparticipants indicated that Teen Outreach was associated with 16% fewer course failures, 23% fewer school suspensions, and 41% fewer pregnancies over the course of a single school year (Allen et al., 1994). The success of Teen Outreach indicates that it is possible to prevent teenage pregnancy without emphasizing sex education. Apparently, the program's effort at increasing teens' educational and vocational aspirations helps youth both avoid pregnancy and do better in school.

School-based or school-linked health clinics have become a popular approach to offering a range of medical, mental health, and health education services to adolescents. The first school-based clinic opened in 1970, and by 1995, over 600 adolescent health clinics had been organized, primarily in low-income communities (Dryfoos, 1995). Because school clinics also provide family planning services, they have been viewed as one possible way to reduce teenage pregnancy. Although statistics indicate that adolescents do utilize services provided by school-based or school-linked clinics, the data have been inconsistent in terms of whether pregnancy rates have been affected (Christopher, 1995).

One program that has been successful, however, is the Self Center, a storefront health clinic located near a junior high and a senior high school in the inner city of Baltimore (Zabin et al., 1986). A multidisciplinary staff consisting of social workers, nurses, and physicians offered health education, personal counseling, and medical services, including contraception. Both formal and informal group education and discussion sessions occurred frequently at the center and at school. Student staff were also recruited to represent the center and to help conduct some of its activities. The center was well received by students. Utilization data indicated that 85% of all students made use of at least one service and students averaged ten contacts. Over a 3-year period the Center was effective in delaying the onset of sexual activity among virgin females and increasing the use of contraception among sexually active youth. Most importantly, substantial changes in pregnancy rates were achieved. Whereas the pregnancy rate declined 30% in the program schools, it rose 58% in control schools.

SUMMARY

Poor physical health places children at risk for social, psychological, and academic problems and creates stress and burdens for caregivers. Several programs have reduced the occurrence of later physical problems and improved physical health. This chapter provided examples of successful interventions conducted at three developmental periods: during infancy and the preschool period, the elementary school years, and adolescence. Programs in the first category suggest the importance of three strategies: (1) a focus on low-income families who are at highest risk for physical health problems; (2) offering multiple services to both adult and child family members; and (3) providing early, intensive, individualized interventions.

Successful programs for school-aged children offer two important lessons: (1) children need to be carefully trained and reinforced if they are to develop new health-related skills, and (2) intervention often needs to move beyond classroom instruction to modify environmental factors that influence health practices. In the latter case, parent and peer involvement and systemic changes in the school curricula and food service have significantly improved children's physical health.

Finally it is possible to prevent adolescent pregnancy, reduce subsequent rates of sexual activity, and teach youth how to protect themselves against HIV/AIDS infection. Once again, systematic skill training is necessary to teach adolescents sex-related behavior (e.g., either how to resist peer pressure and refrain from sexual intercourse or how to have safe sex). Information alone does not produce consistent changes in adolescent sexual behaviors. Furthermore, programs focusing on sexuality must take into consideration parental influences, peer behavior, and social and community norms.

6

Injury Prevention

INTRODUCTION

Physical injuries sustained by children and adolescents are a serious problem involving, quite literally, matters of life and death. At least 10,000 children die each year from unintentional injuries that account for more than 50% of all deaths to children ages 1 to 14, more than the other six major causes of death to children combined (Wilson, Baker, Teret, Shock, & Garbarino, 1991). Moreover, for every death there are an estimated 34 children hospitalized for the treatment of injury, and for every hospitalization, there are 30 more children seen at emergency medical settings. These figures do not include those children treated by private physicians and at home for various injuries. All told, it is believed that every year one out of every five children in the United States suffers an injury requiring some medical attention (Wilson et al., 1991).

Physical injuries can have serious academic, social, and mental health repercussions. Over 30,000 children suffer permanent disabilities of one form or another as a result of injuries annually (Rodriguez, 1990), and children with preexisting physical disabilities are at higher risk than their peers for a variety of social and mental health problems (Lavigne & Faier-Routman, 1992). Injuries to the brain and nervous system can produce enduring negative effects on children's cognitive functioning. Finally, family relationships and functioning can be negatively affected by the need to care for children with chronic conditions.

Furthermore, injuries are extremely costly in both monetary and nonmonetary terms. As already noted, the loss of human life is staggering, and the financial costs of nonfatal injuries are also high. More money is spent treating injuries than on any other childhood medical condition (Miller & Galbraith, 1995). Because injuries disproportionately affect the young, injuries account for more years of potential life lost than cancer and cardiovascular disease combined (National Committee for Injury Prevention and Control, 1989). Last but not least, the emotional pain and suffering of injured parties and their family members should be included in any analysis of injury costs.

Injury prevention and control have never occupied a prominent place in the public agenda. Governmental and social institutions have often failed to take effective action, and much of the general public remains oblivious to the extent of the problem and what can be accomplished. In the mid-1960s, a report prepared by the National Academy of Sciences indicated that injuries were a major problem in the United States but were being neglected; the same organization echoed this lament 20 years later, and emphasized that "Injury is the principal public health problem in America today" (National Academy of Sciences, 1985, p. v).

Although sufficient resources have never been devoted to the injury field, there is room for optimism. Injuries can be prevented. The general public still thinks in terms of "accidents," but workers in the field now use the term *unintentional injury*. In contrast to the view that accidents are unpredictable and "just happen," current research clearly indicates that childhood injuries can be prevented. Wilson et al. (1991) concluded that "... many injuries can be prevented, that children need not be subjected to disability, and that childhood death from injury often reflects a failure to apply existing knowledge and technology" (p. 231).

Additional Facts about Injury

Table 6.1 summarizes additional facts about specific types of injuries affecting youth. The risk for different types of injuries varies with the age of the child and illustrates the importance of a developmental perspective. Injury risk is high in infancy due to falls, motor vehicle crashes, and asphyxiation; preschoolers are at high risk for fire, burn, and pedestrian injuries; risk is highest among the elementary school years for pedestrian injuries; and adolescents are at high risk when driving motor vehicles and for drowning. In general, males are twice as likely as females to incur injuries.

The different injuries affecting youth at different ages means that specific interventions may work for one type of injury for one age group but not for other injuries affecting younger or older children. Finally, it should be noted that few lend any credence to the once-held view of an "accident-prone personality style" (Rivara & Mueller, 1987). Risky behaviors, inadequate adult supervision, and environmental circumstances seem to be the major determinants of injury.

Table 6.1. Statistics on Major Types of Childhood Injuries

Type of injury	General information
Pedestrian injuries	Leading cause of death, ages 4–8; for all ages, 80,000 injuries; 1,100 deaths caused in traffic situations and 200 more in driveways and parking lots
Fires and burns	House fires kill about 1,200; 100,000 children are treated for burns due to scalding hot water
Bicycles	Highest cause of injury next to automobiles; 400 killed and 400,000 require emergency treatment annually
Poisoning	About 700,000 nonfatal poisonings a year concentrated in those under 5
Falls	Leading cause of nonfatal injury; as many as 9,000 falls from cribs, 8,000 from high chairs, and 22,000 from bunk beds; falls account for one third of all hospital admissions for head injury and one third of all emergency visits
Motor vehicles	7,800 deaths among drivers under age 20 in 1992; as passengers, 1,600 deaths among those under 15 and more than 200,000 nonfatal injuries
Other vehicles	Minibikes, mopeds, and trail bikes account for about 13,000 injuries; snowmobiles and all-terrain vehicles for an additional 38,000
Firearms	In 1992, 784 children 0 to 14 and 9,463 adolescents and young adults died from firearms; among those 16 or younger, half of handgun injuries occurred at home
Playgrounds and sports	Few deaths but many injuries: 170,000 injuries associated with playground equipment; 600,000 related to sports and recreation
Drowning	2,000 drownings among those less than 19; a major cause of death among 1 to 4 year olds
Home accidents	Approximately 11 out of every 100 children less than 4 years old and 9 out of every 100 between 5 and 17 are injured in home accidents of various kinds

Note: All data are annual figures and are drawn from Wilson et al. (1991) and the National Safety Council (1993).

Approaches to Injury Prevention

The different conceptual frameworks that have been advanced in the injury field can be translated into the conceptual model used throughout this book. In other words, programs to prevent childhood injury can occur at either the individual or the environmental level. The intervention can target all children in a population, those considered to be at highest risk and occasionally those undergoing important life transitions.

Some within the injury field believe that redesign of the physical environment and legislation are the most effective intervention strategies; others point out that such strategies are not applicable or helpful in all circumstances. Several sources summarize the pros and cons of these positions (Baker, 1981; Finney et al., 1993; Peterson & Roberts, 1992; Roberts, 1987; Robertson, 1983). It appears that no single approach is effective in all situations. In the following two major sections, representative interventions occurring at the environmental and individual level are described.

ENVIRONMENTAL INTERVENTIONS

Effects of Legislation

Legislation regulating product redesign has been particularly effective in reducing certain types of injuries. For example, legislation requiring the manufacturing of flame-retardant sleepwear for young children has reduced the number of fire-related injuries (Smith & Falk, 1987), and the Refrigerator Safety Act, which banned products that could not be opened from the inside, has almost completely eliminated children's deaths from asphyxiation when trapped in refrigerators (Robertson, 1983).

Walton (1982) has described the very positive impact of the Poison Prevention Packaging Act (PPPA) of 1970. PPPA requires that potentially hazardous household substances be sold in special packaging that is difficult for children under the age of 5 to open (so-called child-proof packages). Fifteen different regulations covering various products such as aspirin, paint solvent, and prescription drugs eventually emerged from the original legislation. Walton (1982) estimated that from 1973 to 1978, safety packaging legislation resulted in a fourfold decrease in the poisoning death rate among young children and saved approximately 300 lives each year. During this same time period, over 193,750 fatal and nonfatal poisonings were prevented.

Legislation relative to other aspects of injury control may have some impact, but additional methods are needed to change behavior. This is the case with respect to the use of car safety devices (CSD) for infants and young children. There is a strong relationship between the use of CSDs and injuries and death. Children not in CSDs are 11 times more likely to die in motor vehicle crashes than those in such devices (Decker, Dewey, Hutcheson, & Shafner, 1984). Accordingly, it has been estimated that up to 70% of all serious automobile-related injuries and up to 90% of child fatalities could be avoided through the use of CSDs (Roberts & Turner, 1984). Currently, all states and the District of Columbia have laws requiring the use of CSDs, but legislation by itself does not insure compliance. One 3-year study conducted in five states indicated that following passage of new legislation requiring the use of CSDs, compliance increased sharply in two states, stayed the same in one, and decreased in two others (Seekins et al., 1988). Several behaviorally oriented community-based interventions that have been successful in increasing the use of CSDs (Roberts & Turner, 1984) are described below.

Child Car Safety Devices

Roberts and his colleagues have conducted a series of interventions to increase the use of CSDs (summarized in Roberts, Layfield & Fanurik, 1992). The general approach has been to use relatively inexpensive incentives (e.g., stickers, coloring books, and lottery tickets good for free pizza) to reward children who are in safety seats when being driven to child care centers or elementary schools. The impact of these programs was evaluated by observing the percentage of cars in which all occupants (not just the child passenger) are observed using seat belts or car seats appropriately. Observations are taken during a baseline phase, during the intervention when incentives are offered, and then at follow-up when incentives are removed.

Findings from six separate studies have been combined and are presented in Fig. 6.1. The six interventions did significantly change safety behavior. The percentage of cars in which all occupants were using safety restraints correctly averaged 21% at baseline, 68% during the reward condition, and 44% during follow-up periods that ranged from 2 to 18 weeks. In other words, although there was some loss of effect over time, the percentage of cars in which all occupants were using appropriate seat restraints at follow-up still represented a 109% increase over baseline levels.

The program reported by Roberts, Fanurik, and Wilson (1988) illustrates the application of this intervention on a large-scale community-wide basis. Twenty-five elementary schools serving 9000 children in the metropolitan area of Tuscaloosa, Alabama participated. Community resources were mobilized to support and conduct this program. For instance, a pizza company provided funding for the major incentives, local media popularized the program by running announcements and news stories, and members of the schools' PTA and older children who were part of the school safety patrol helped implement the intervention.

To assess the impact of the program, observers recorded whether each vehicle occupant (adult *and* child) arriving at school each morning was buckled up properly. During the incentive phase of the program, children riding in CSDs received stickers, bumper stickers, or lottery tickets good for a drawing for a free family dinner at a local restaurant.

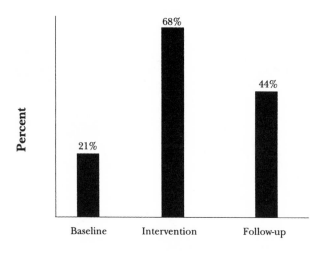

Figure 6.1. Percentage of cars in which occupants are using adult seat beats and child safety seats. Data are averaged across six studies described by Roberts, Layfield, and Fanurik (1992).

Incentives ceased after 3 weeks of the reward condition and observations of vehicles continued for 2 weeks of follow-up. Results were consistent with the other studies conducted by Roberts and his colleagues. At baseline, all occupants were using CSDs appropriately in only 18% of observed vehicles; during the intervention this percentage increased almost fourfold to 65% and dropped to 49% during follow-up, which was still a 272% increase over baseline levels.

There are several interesting features to the Roberts et al. (1988) intervention. First is the demonstration of how community resources can be mobilized to support child safety programs. Second, program contingencies modified adult as well as child safety behavior, since children could receive rewards only if adults were also using seat belts. Third, although a complete analysis was not conducted, the intervention seemed cost-effective. The financial contribution from the local business was returned through the free advertising that was generated by the program, and PTA members volunteered their time to implement the intervention. Finally, Roberts and his colleagues have noted that some parents steadfastly refused to participate in their safety program, suggesting that further efforts are needed to motivate the hard-to-reach (unresponsive) members of the population.

Wearing of Bicycle Helmets

The situation with respect to bicycle helmets is similar to that of CSDs. Wearing bicycle helmets can reduce injuries. For instance, over 500 young people under the age of 20 die from bicycle-related injuries each year; injuries to the head are the primary cause in up to 80% of these deaths, and bicycle helmets can prevent up to 85% of head and brain injuries (Bergman, Rivara, Richards, & Rogers, 1990). Yet, most children who ride bicycles do not wear helmets; studies often report figures of less than 10%. In summary, the most effective way to prevent serious injuries to bicycle riders is to increase the consistent use of bicycle helmets. What is the best way to achieve this goal? Two general approaches have been tried: traditional education and multifaceted community promotion campaigns; the latter have been much more successful than the former.

For example, in Seattle, Washington, a community coalition involving the schools, health departments, local media, and businesses was successful in tripling the rate of children who wore bicycle helmets from 5% to 16% over a 16-month period; there were essentially no changes observed in a control community (Bergman et al., 1990). Extending the program for 2 more years increased the use of bicycle helmets to 38% (Thompson, Thompson, Rivara, & Salazar, 1993). Similar communitywide promotional programs conducted outside the United States have reported similar results. Bicycle helmet use by children rose from 4.6% to 38.6% in Australia (Wood & Milne, 1988) and from 1.3% to 33% in Quebec, Canada (Farley, Haddad, & Brown, 1995).

It is particularly important to give community promotional programs sufficient time to exert their effects before reaching any conclusions, because changing social norms and behavior takes time. For instance, after 1 year of intervention, bicycle helmet use was only around 10% in the above community programs, but this rate eventually tripled over the next few years.

One research group (Cote et al., 1992; Dannenberg, Gielen, Beilenson, Wison, & Joffe, 1993) evaluated the impact of the first bicycle helmet law passed in the United States. In 1990, a law was passed in Howard County, Maryland, requiring all those under the age of 16 to wear an approved safety helmet when riding a bicycle. This legislation was accompanied by an extensive community promotion campaign to encourage the purchase and use of bicycle helmets. The effect of the new law and community campaign was evaluated using two surrounding counties. In one of these comparison counties there had been a community promotion effort to increase helmet use but no legislation, and in the other there was neither legislation nor an educational campaign.

Legislation combined with a community campaign in Howard County was most effective in increasing use of bicycle helmets (from 4% at pretest to 47% at posttest). The promotional campaign alone increased helmet use from 8% to 19%, and there was no change over time in the county in which neither legislation nor education was attempted. The magnitude of change occurring in Howard County was thus substantial, but it is important to note that more than half of targeted children were still not wearing helmets.

Although some injury interventions are sometimes referred to as investigating the effects of "education" or "legislation" (e.g., Bergman et al., 1990; Cote et al., 1992), these terms are misleading. Both of these programs, as well as the others discussed above, included many components in addition to education or legislation. The activities of multiple community organizations were carefully coordinated. Bicycle fairs and other community events were held to promote social norms favoring helmet use and featured opportunities for children to see helmet use modeled by peers and adults. Discounts for purchasing helmets were offered to families and children were also rewarded for wearing helmets. The Canadian program (Farley et al., 1995), for instance, involved the cooperation of teachers, police officers, retailers, recreation departments, and organizers of sporting events; over 250 different agencies participated each year. Therefore, I have used the term *community promotion campaign* to describe these interventions. In contrast, when education has been the predominant intervention strategy, programs have not been effective in increasing the wearing of bicycle helmets (Cushman, James, & Waclawik, 1991; Pendergrast, Ashworth, DuRant, & Litaker, 1992).

Prevention of Other Types of Injuries

The same two approaches—education and community promotion campaigns—have also been used to prevent other types of injuries with similar results. Educational approaches have been called "lecture and pamphlet programs" (Pless & Arsenault, 1987) to reflect that the main components of such programs usually consist of a brief didactic presentation along with the distribution of educational literature that recommends taking some action. Although lecture and pamphlet programs are continually being conducted by hospitals, various community settings, schools, and occasionally through the media, evidence is lacking that such programs are effective in reducing injuries or increasing safety behaviors. Consistent with other areas of prevention (such as AIDS and sex education, pregnancy prevention, and substance use), devoting time and energy to an exclusive educational approach toward prevention is misguided. Merely educating people regarding the need to prevent injuries does not change their behavior. In contrast, several community promotion programs have achieved positive results. Table 6.2 summarizes the general characteristics and results of four successful programs that are discussed in more detail below.

The Children Can't Fly program (Spiegel & Lindaman, 1977) originated from two events. The first was the finding from an epidemiological study indicating that an unusually high number of children were dying from falls out of high-rise apartment buildings in New York City, particularly in the South Bronx. These results prompted the second event, which was an ordinance passed in 1976 by the New York City Board of Health requiring owners of multiple dwellings to provide window guards in apartments where children younger than age 10 resided. Although the Children Can't Fly Program is sometimes cited as an example of the impact of legislation and environmental redesign on injury prevention, the intervention was more complicated than that.

A community coalition composed of health care agencies, schools, tenant groups, and churches was created to convince residents of the need for action to prevent injuries from falls. In the most important aspect of the program, outreach workers made door-to-door visits to apartments to teach parents how to install and use window guards. The window guards were distributed free-of-charge to all families who requested them. Outreach workers installed the window guards if requested, but 75% were installed by the apartment residents themselves (and not by the landlords, who were culpable according to the new law). The intervention produced a dramatic 31% decline in the incidence of all falls throughout New York City and a 50% decline in the South Bronx area, where such falls had been most frequent. There was also a 35% citywide drop in deaths of young children due to falls over a 2-year period.

Schelp (1987, 1988) has described a comprehensive approach to injury prevention in rural Sweden that represents another collaborative undertaking between health officials and local citizens. A large community coalition was formed that eventually involved over 60 different agencies and community groups. Health officials and citizen groups worked collectively to identify needs and priorities, plan programs, and collect data. As a result, many citizens became actively involved in promoting safety.

Safety training programs were created in the schools and at child

Table 6.2. Some Exemplary Community-Based Injury Prevention Programs

Program	Main goals	Intervention components	Primary outcomes
Davidson et al. (1994)	Injuries from vehicles, falls, and guns	Community coalition organized various programs; repair playground equipment, safety training, improve adult supervision at sporting events	26% reduction in injuries
Schelp (1987)	All types of home injuries	Community coalition organized many programs; safety training in home and school; free safety products	33% reduction in injuries
Schwartz et al. (1993)	Falls, scald burns, assaults, gun injuries	Community residents implement the program; home safety inspections, free safety products	Experimental homes enacted more safety measures
Spiegel & Lindaman (1977)	Falls from windows	Community coalition; home inspections, free window guard	50% reduction in all falls; 35% reduction in deaths

and health agencies. Safety consciousness was kept high in the community by rotating exhibits and demonstrations through many different settings such as pharmacies, banks, and libraries. Local businesses also cooperated by selling safety products promoted in the exhibits. Safety training was also conducted through home visits that were coordinated with pediatric health services. Finally, safety equipment such as infant car seats and life vests were distributed free of charge based on need. The Swedish program was particularly successful in reducing child and adolescent injuries. There was a 33% reduction in the overall incidence of children's home injuries and a 20% reduction in injuries among adolescents and young adults (ages 15–24) over a 3-year period.

The Safe Kids/Healthy Neighborhoods Program (SKHN) (Davidson et al., 1994) is another example of a community coalition approach to injury prevention. SKHN was formed in the Harlem community of New York City to combat the high rates of injuries occurring among children in that community. Overall, 26 organizations, including local health departments, schools, voluntary organizations, and community groups, cooperated in a multifaceted program. The coalition organized efforts to repair playground equipment, to conduct an intensive pedestrian safety training program, to improve adult supervision of sports and recreational activities, and to promote the use of bicycle helmets. Similar to the Swedish program (Schelp, 1987, 1988), several program components were developed based on local citizens' expressed needs and priorities.

An injury surveillance system monitored the occurrence of serious pediatric injuries resulting in hospitalization or death. Compared to 6 years of preintervention data, SKHN produced a 26% reduction in serious injuries over a 3-year period in the targeted age group (children 5 to 16 years old).

Finally, the Safe Block Project (SBP) (Schwartz, Grisso, Miles, Holmes, & Sutton, 1993) represents another successful attempt at involving local citizens in injury prevention. SBP focused on a low-income urban community in Philadelphia populated largely by African Americans and that had high rates of home injuries. SBP employed an innovative three-tier staffing arrangement. Research staff hired, trained, and then supervised 13 residents from the community who served as community liaisons or home safety inspectors. The community liaisons were responsible, in turn, for recruiting volunteer block leaders to assist in program implementation. The block leaders contacted families residing on their blocks and conducted monthly safety meetings to educate their neighbors in specific safety topics and to prompt appropriate behavioral changes. Participation rates were high. Volunteer block leaders were successfully recruited for 88% of the target blocks, and only 9% of the families who were subsequently approached for the home safety program declined to participate.

The prime element of the intervention consisted of a systematic home safety inspection. These inspections evaluated home safety features, taught household members how to correct safety hazards, and provided free supplies as needed (e.g., smoke detectors and batteries, a bathwater thermometer for scald burn prevention, and so on). The cost of these safety supplies averaged only $10.34 per home. Additional home features that were examined included frayed electrical wiring, proper storage and labeling of medications, presence of peeling paint, broken steps and railings, tripping hazards, and storage of weapons.

After a year-long intervention, another home safety inspection was conducted to evaluate the program. The program was effective in changing several home safety behaviors. For instance, compared to homes in control communities, intervention homes were seven times more likely to have a poison emetic on hand (e.g., syrup of ipecac, which induces vomiting if a child ingests a hazardous substance), twice as likely to have a fire escape plan, 19% more likely to have a working smoking detector, and 16% more likely to keep medicines out of reach of children. However, few differences were observed in those safety features that required the most effort to modify such as broken steps, loose railings, and peeling paint.

Elements of Effective Community Programs

The studies listed in Table 6.2 are impressive in terms of their planning, execution, and outcomes. These programs seem to have made a real difference in children's lives by significantly reducing death and injury. Furthermore, they have been successful in rural and urban settings and for white and nonwhite populations. Because each intervention has multiple elements, it is not possible to identify exactly which program features have been responsible for outcomes. Nevertheless, successful programs share several common features that could be profitably emulated by others.

First, specific program objectives are established that are informed by previous research or locally obtained epidemiological data. This scientific grounding is important for program planning by identifying what types of injuries are occurring, where, and who is most affected. Second, to insure broad public support, community coalitions are formed involving as many local agencies and citizen groups as possible. In a true spirit of collaboration, coalition members share responsibility for various aspects of program planning and execution. Coalition building provides several potential benefits such as insuring that local needs and priorities are addressed and that the community has a stronger commitment to the program once it is begun.

Third, when many community members participate in multiple activities over time, social norms promoting injury prevention are likely to be enhanced. Considering the public's usual low level of awareness regarding the need for injury prevention, modifying relevant social norms can be an important long-term benefit. Fourth, the home-based nature of many programs seems critical. Families given home demonstrations and training are in a better position to take the necessary steps to change because the intervention is individualized to suit their unique living arrangements. In other words, the intervention has a high degree of ecological validity. Finally, providing incentives for behavioral change in the form of free or steeply discounted safety products also seems helpful.

INDIVIDUAL LEVEL INTERVENTIONS

Training Children in Safety Behaviors

Several interventions have successfully used behavioral procedures to teach children various safety skills. The procedures typically involve modeling, practice, and reinforcement, and children have learned how to avoid strangers, escape fires, and cross streets safely (see Roberts, Fanurik, & Layfield, 1987). Although these programs have been effective, they are usually labor intensive and involve small samples. More programs are needed to reach children in a more economical fashion such as the approach taken by Yeaton and Bailey (1983).

After first demonstrating that procedures were effective in directly teaching 24 young children pedestrian safety skills, Yeaton and Bailey (1983) extended their intervention to over 500 kindergarten and first graders attending nine different schools. Their approach consisted of first training adult crossing guards employed at the schools, who, in turn, successfully taught the children how to cross streets safely. Using videotapes and role-playing procedures, it only took one training session for guards to acquire the necessary training skills. As the children journeyed back and forth to school, the crossing guards instructed them on how to cross streets safely. As a result of training, the children showed dramatic gains in their performance over time and were observed to be crossing the street safely over 90% of the time.

Training key adults in the school environment can greatly increase the child population that is served over the long run. For instance, once school crossing guards attain the necessary training competence, they remain in a position to help each new wave of children entering their respective schools year after year.

Latchkey Children

Other programs are examples of targeting high-risk groups for injury prevention. Peterson and her group have concentrated on latchkey children who are at particularly high risk for injury, because by definition latchkey children are without adult supervision for varying periods of the day. Therefore, these children must be capable of dealing with numerous potentially risky situations such as handling strangers, operating home appliances, and preparing food. Peterson's group has been very successful in helping children acquire multiple safety behaviors either by working directly with the children or through their teachers and parents. Furthermore, the trained children often maintain most of their gains during follow-up (see Peterson, 1989, for a summary).

As an example of this work, two groups of parents were supervised on how to teach their children various safety skills. (Peterson, Mori, Selby, & Rosen, 1988). Training manuals were given to parents and their children. Each week one group of parents met for 1 hour to receive supervision, while the other group was given consultation over the phone. Nine safety behaviors divided into three main areas were targeted. These included everyday happenings (e.g., preparing food), emergencies (e.g., treating burns or cuts), and strangers (e.g., dealing with strangers at the door, outside, or on the phone). The children in both parent conditions learned the safety skills, and a 6-month follow-up assessment indicated that most children continued to demonstrate near-perfect performance on most of the targeted skills.

There are several important lessons to be learned from these studies. First, the need is great for safety training. Data clearly indicate that most latchkey children are unable to perform almost all safety behaviors adequately without systematic training. Furthermore, almost all parents overestimate their child's ability to handle potentially risky situations, while they underestimate the possibility of many types of injury. In reference to latchkey children, Peterson (1989) observed: "The easiest summary statement is that they did not know a fraction of what they needed to know or what their parents typically believed they know" (p. 40).

Second, effective training must provide children with sufficient opportunity to practice and to obtain feedback. Such training is labor-intensive but necessary to achieve mastery. Children must learn the skills to the point that they become habitual and this takes time. Third, to insure maintenance of new skills, booster training sessions are recommended, particularly for behaviors not frequently used (e.g., exiting a fire or attending to a burn). Fourth, parents' willingness to follow a systematic program tends to wax and wane over time, and consistent encouragement is often needed to maintain their motivation. Social and at times physical reinforcement (such as stickers or charts) are also helpful to solidify children's skill development. Fifth, the number of parents who are willing to conduct safety training for their children is not known, and the participation of some parents may be very difficult to obtain. Nevertheless, for some populations, such as latchkey children, direct training of safety behaviors may be the only feasible approach.

Interventions by Physicians

Physicians, particularly pediatricians, can play an important role in injury prevention. A review of 20 programs indicates that office-based counseling conducted by physicians or their staff is an effective strategy in injury prevention, and that preventive activities can be integrated into routine medical practice (Bass et al., 1993). Office-based counseling does not always reduce injuries or increase safety behavior, however. The likelihood of success seems to increase when the intervention is developmentally appropriate, extends over multiple rather than single appointments, makes safety products easily available and at reduced cost, and is part of a larger community-based effort to reduce injuries. The United States Preventive Services Task Force (1989) and the American Academy of Pediatrics (see Bass et al., 1993) have recognized injury prevention as an effective intervention and have recommended its incorporation into routine pediatric health care.

SUMMARY

A review of injury prevention efforts suggests, first of all, that success is possible. The rate of fatal and nonfatal injuries sustained by children can be reduced, sometimes substantially. Lives have been saved and the negative consequences that are likely to follow serious nonfatal injuries can be prevented. This is very encouraging.

Second, it appears that different approaches are effective, depending on the circumstances. Legislation and regulation have been particularly effective in terms of designing safer products (e.g., infant sleep-wear and safety packaging for hazardous household products). Legislation also has some positive effect on other behaviors such as the use of car safety seats and bicycle helmets, but additional tactics usually must be used to increase compliance in these areas. The use of incentives and social reinforcement, or these techniques used within a broad community promotion campaign, seem to be effective in substantially increasing the use of car and bicycle safety products.

In those cases where legislation is not practical, approaches to train children in safety behaviors have met with success. Some children at high risk for potential injury, such as latchkey children, have been well served by these interventions. Several effective community-oriented programs have focused on home safety. These multifaceted programs are often characterized by community organization and coalition building, intervention in the home, and financial incentives to facilitate behavioral change.

Although several programs have changed safety behaviors or injury rates, there is still much room for improvement. Many children and adolescents are still experiencing unnecessary injuries that can have negative long-term effects on their adjustment. Hopefully, the successes that have been obtained in injury prevention will encourage further research and practice. The decision to include a separate chapter on injuries in this book was based on the view that this topic deserves as much attention as any other in the prevention area. Furthermore, some approaches in injury prevention, such as broad-based community promotion programs and the use of community coalitions, can serve as useful models for interventions in other areas of children's lives such as mental health, child maltreatment, and physical health promotion.

7

Child Maltreatment

INTRODUCTION

Maltreatment is a general term that encompasses neglect and physical, sexual, and emotional abuse. Many children are maltreated. In 1994, there were more than one million confirmed cases of abuse and neglect (Children's Defense Fund, 1995). Due to a lack of precision in its definition plus the reluctance to report or confirm abuse, the true incidence may be two to three times higher than official figures suggest.

Consequences of Maltreatment

Maltreatment tends to have a variety of serious short- and long-term effects. The most serious is loss of life. Between 1200 to 1500 deaths result from physical abuse and neglect each year (Willis, Holden, & Rosenberg, 1992). Severe physical abuse can result in lasting physiological damage. During childhood, physical abuse is associated with a variety of emotional, behavioral, and academic problems. Over the longer term, physical abuse is related to externalizing, criminal, and self-injurious behavior during adolescence and more adult forms of violence toward dating partners and spouses. Maltreated children are also more likely to become victims of violence or abuse in adulthood (Malinosky-Rummell & Hansen, 1993).

Many different childhood emotional and behavioral problems can also occur following sexual abuse. A frequent clinical diagnosis is post-traumatic stress disorder (Kendall-Tackett, Williams, & Finkelhor, 1993). In adulthood, lowered self-esteem and heightened anxiety and depression have been found (Jumper, 1995). Some studies also suggest that sexually abused children of both genders are at risk for impaired sexual functioning during adulthood.

One particularly pernicious effect of maltreatment is its intergenerational character. Those who are maltreated in childhood are more likely to maltreat their children. Thus, the cycle of maltreatment continues into the next generation. It is no longer believed that all parents who abuse their children were abused when they were children, although the factors responsible for the continuation of abuse across generations are unknown. Experts now suggest that 30% (plus or minus 5%) of parents who maltreat their children received similar treatment when they were children (Kaufman & Zigler, 1987; Widom, 1989).

In summary, the problem of child maltreatment is widespread and can have many serious repercussions. Prevention is important because of the limited success achieved in treating abuse once it occurs. One review of 89 funded demonstration projects primarily targeting physical abuse and neglect (Cohn & Daro, 1987) indicated that a relatively high percentage of parents (30–47%) continued to abuse their children *while in treatment* and over 50% were judged likely to abuse after treatment termination. A more recent review uncovered few indications that treatment reduces subsequent abuse (Oates & Bross, 1995). Furthermore, physically abusive families are difficult to engage in treatment and dropout rates are high. After reviewing interventions for abusive families, Wolfe and Wekerle (1993) concluded that preventive approaches are likely to be more practical and cost-effective than treatment of physical abuse and neglect after the fact.

Treatment for sexual abuse is also difficult because many cases go unreported and many families deny the existence of the problem. It has been estimated that treatment occurs in only one out of eight families in which sexual abuse occurs (Alter-Reid, Gibbs, Lachenmeyer, Sigal, & Massoth, 1986). This figure is probably increasing as more attention is being devoted to sexual abuse. Nevertheless, many instances of sexual abuse are not discovered until long after the abuse has occurred.

In the following sections, programs attempting primary prevention of physical abuse, neglect, and sexual abuse are discussed, and then a few secondary prevention programs in these areas are reviewed.

PHYSICAL ABUSE AND NEGLECT

Risk and Protective Factors

Both physical abuse and neglect are multiply determined and a risk and protective factor paradigm provides a useful perspective for viewing preventive interventions:

There not only appears to be no single cause of child maltreatment, but no necessary or sufficient causes. All too sadly, there are many pathways to child abuse and neglect.... Moreover, it is well appreciated that what determines whether child maltreatment will take place is the balance of stressors and supports or of potentiating (i.e., risk) and compensatory (i.e., protective) factors. (Belsky, 1993, p. 413)

Table 7.1 lists risk factors at the community–social, parental, and child level that have been associated with physical abuse. Some child factors are listed in Table 7.1, not to suggest that children are in any way to blame for abuse, but to indicate that by virtue of their physical condition, temperament, or behavior, some children are at greater risk for abuse than others.

Families are often besieged by an accumulation of the risk factors noted in Table 7.1. For instance, the child-abusing parent is often socially isolated, under extreme economic and social pressure, and may have personal problems involving depression or substance abuse. Furthermore, abusive parents often hold unrealistic expectations about child development and become frustrated or angry when their children do not meet these expectations. Abusive parents do not perceive their children as responsive or very rewarding, and thus derive little satisfaction from parenting. Finally, parents are highly stressed by a variety of personal, familial, and social factors. Parental frustration and anger-

Table 7.1. Prominent Risk Factors
Related to Child Physical Abuse and Neglect

Community and social factors
1. Social norms
   a. High tolerance of violence
   b. Acceptance of physical punishment to control behavior
   c. Mass media portrayals of violence
   d. Preeminence of parental "rights" (ownership of children)
2. Social impoverishment: communities characterized by crime, high mobility, few services, and a negative or poor sense of community
3. High stress: resulting from economic and social factors

Parental factors
1. Demographics: young, single, low-income, large family size
2. History of childhood abuse
3. Personal problems: substance abuse, depression, difficulty in controlling negative emotions
4. Unplanned pregnancy
5. Child-rearing practices: unrealistic expectations, punitive discipline practices
6. High stress: resulting from personal, marital, or family factors

Child factors
1. Physical factors: health problems, developmental disabilities
2. Behavioral factors: difficult temperament, noncompliance

Note: This information is drawn primarily from Belsky (1993) and Peterson and Brown (1994).

builds over time and their interactions with their children become successively more punitive and ultimately abusive.

The ecology of abuse often requires that multiple services be provided. Interventions attempt to prevent abuse by providing social support to alleviate parental isolation and stress, by helping parents secure needed psychological and health services for themselves and their family members, and by promoting effective child-rearing practices. In the latter case, the general goal is to foster a positive parent–child relationship, which should protect against maltreatment. In preventive programs, parents frequently learn about infant and child development and how to respond appropriately to child behaviors and manage everyday child care tasks. Services are usually provided in home visits that occur on a regular basis and whose elements can be individualized to suit each family's needs. Many programs use a high-risk approach in selecting populations for intervention and have focused on low-income, young, and unmarried mothers. Although there have not been many controlled empirical evaluations of programs to prevent child abuse, positive findings have appeared in a few well-conducted studies (MacMillan, MacMillan, Offord, Griffith, & MacMillan, 1994a).

Representative Programs

Olds, Henderson, Chamberlin, and Tatelbaum (1986) studied a large sample of white, first-time mothers characterized by one or more of the following three risk factors: under 19 years of age, single parents, and low-income status. Two home-visiting interventions that began during the 30th week of the mother's pregnancy and varied in intensity and duration were evaluated along with an untreated control group. In the first treatment condition, mothers were visited until the child's birth, whereas in the other treatment group mothers received continuing visits until the child was 2 years of age. The home visits had two primary goals: (1) to promote mothers' ability to understand and respond to their children's needs, and (2) to increase the social support received by the mother. In the latter case, home visitors provided direct support to mothers and helped them secure additional support from friends, relatives, and neighbors.

The intervention positively affected the parent–child relationship and resulted in better child outcomes; in general, the more intensive intervention was more effective. For instance, mothers reported less conflict with their babies and viewed them as having more positive moods and crying less frequently. In addition, nurse visitors' observations indicated that mothers provided more appropriate play materials and restricted or punished their children less often. Home visitation that continued through the first 2 years of the child's life resulted in fewer visits to the emergency rooms of local hospitals and fewer cases of accidents and poisonings. Most importantly, the rate of child abuse for the sample of mothers who possessed all three of the risk factors (i.e., for the young, low-income, unmarried mothers) was almost five times lower than for controls (4% versus 19%, respectively). In other words, this program produced a substantial reduction in child abuse for the group at greatest risk.

A 2-year follow-up conducted when the children were approximately 4 years old (Olds, Henderson, & Kitzman, 1994) failed to find a significant difference in rates of maltreatment between the intensive home-visiting intervention and controls. Most other outcome variables, however, suggested that the children in the nurse-visited families were receiving better care. For instance, nurse-visited children had experienced 40% fewer injuries and ingestions of hazardous substances, had been brought to medical emergency departments 35% fewer times, and had 45% fewer behavioral problems according to parent reports. The homes of nurse-visited families were also evaluated as containing more safety features.

Hardy and Street (1989) evaluated a similar home-visiting program that also offered mothers child care assistance and social support. In this case, the target group was low-income, inner-city African-American mothers, many of whom (78%) were single. The home visits began when the child was 7 to 10 days old and continued for approximately 2 years as the mother and child completed scheduled appointments at a pediatric clinic.

Several positive outcomes were obtained. First, the rate of child abuse and neglect was six times lower in the experimental than in the control group. Second, experimental mothers were more effective in securing preventive medical care for their children (e.g., 88% of study children vs. 69% of control children had received recommended immunizations). Third, there were one third as many occurrences of major illness or injuries requiring hospitalization among the experimental group. Finally, although a complete cost analysis was not accomplished, the new program seemed to save money compared to no intervention. Analysis of the cost of medical services for the experimental and control groups including the salary of the home visitor indicated that the intervention saved approximately $25,000 over the 24-month program period. This cost savings was conservative, since it did not include the expenses involved in the investigation and management of abuse and neglect that occurred more frequently in the control group.

Although only a few studies provide direct evidence, several additional investigations offer indirect evidence that abuse can be prevented. These other studies come from the literatures on child and maternal health programs, family support and preservation programs, and home-visiting programs. Some of this work was discussed in Chapter 5. These interventions are not traditionally seen as attempts to prevent child maltreatment, but have sought to modify similar risk factors (parental child-rearing practices and high stress), frequently use the same variables to identify families at risk (such as young, low-income mothers), and emphasize a similar strategy in delivering services (namely, home visiting). Several of these interventions have improved parental child-rearing practices and the parent–child relationship, with concomitant benefits observed in children's health and medical status and their social and cognitive development. Although these studies rarely collect outcome data on rates of child maltreatment, authors are beginning to recognize their relevance to child abuse prevention (Wolfe, Reppucci, & Hart, 1995). One cannot conclude definitely that these programs have prevented abuse in the absence of specific outcome data. Nevertheless, because these programs have successfully modified important indices of risk relative to abuse, child maltreatment is less likely to occur.

In summary, conclusions about the prevention of physical abuse and neglect must be offered cautiously for several reasons. First, there is a need for more studies that assess abusive behaviors, follow families over time, and determine how different risk and protective factors operate to influence abuse. Second, most interventions have only collected outcome data on mothers. This is a serious limitation. Males abuse children and their spouses, and the latter can further traumatize children. Between 40 to 60% of males who abuse women also abuse children (American Psychological Association, 1996). Third, physical abuse has been studied more frequently than neglect, although data indicate that the latter form of abuse is more than twice as likely to be officially confirmed (Children's Defense Fund, 1995).

Notwithstanding these limitations, effective programs tend to be most distinctive in terms of what services are offered, to whom, where, and when. Primary prevention of child abuse and neglect seems possible, providing that the intervention is of long duration (generally a year or more), begins before birth or very soon after, involves home-based services, and is focused on populations at risk. Programs that effectively provide social support and strengthen parental child-rearing competencies have been successful. Such services appear to improve the parent–

child relationship, which may serve as a major protective factor against maltreatment.

PREVENTION OF SEXUAL ABUSE

Primary Prevention

In contrast to physical abuse and neglect interventions that have primarily targeted high-risk parents, sexual abuse prevention (SAP) programs have been directed primarily at teaching children about sexual abuse in order to prevent them from being victimized. Children are also taught to report quickly any instances of abuse that occur or are attempted. SAP is a relatively recent phenomenon. The first programs began in the late 1970s, but there are now about 600 SAP programs of one form or another (Kohl, 1993). Despite concerns about the proliferation of untested programs (Reppucci & Haugaard, 1989), most SAP programs have never been subjected to any careful evaluation.

Although programs vary in procedures and goals, McGrath and Bogat (1995) indicate that the aim of many programs for young children can be summarized as Recognition, No, Go, and Tell. That is, programs teach children the difference between good and bad touch (Recognition), and if bad touch occurs, how to be assertive in resisting it (No), leave the situation (Go), and inform a trusted adult about what happened (Tell). Programs for older children generally include the same components and emphasize strategies to resist the attempted victimization. All programs emphasize that abuse is never the child's fault.

Developmentally appropriate curricula must be constructed and evaluated for children at different ages to insure that participants can comprehend the instruction. For instance, discriminating good from bad touches coming from family members, distinguishing intentions from behaviors, and understanding why it is okay to break certain "secrets" are difficult concepts for young children to understand. Reservations have been expressed regarding how well young children can acquire and retain these concepts and use them to protect themselves (Melton, 1992; Wolfe et al., 1995).

There have only been about 30 empirical evaluations of SAP using any types of control groups, and outcome data provide limited evidence for preventive effects (Finkelhor & Strapko, 1992; MacMillan, MacMillan, Offord, Griffith, & MacMillan, 1994b; Wolfe et al., 1995). Researchers usually use proxy variables to assess outcomes. That is, instead of examining rates of future abuse, studies assess if children are more knowledgeable about abuse and more skillful in terms of how to defend themselves. Data do indicate that children do increase their knowledge about abuse and learn skills related to thwarting potential abuse. Older children seem to profit more than younger children, but the latter can also benefit, providing that the training is developmentally appropriate and permits practice and reinforcement of new skills. Overall, however, follow-ups have been limited in number and duration, and in some cases, program effects have diminished over time.

One noteworthy study examining whether SAP programs prevent future abuse has yielded discouraging results. A telephone survey obtained data from a nationally representative sample of 2000 youngsters between the ages of 10 and 16 (Finkelhor, Asdigian, & Dziuba-Leatherman, 1995a) and compared children who did or did not receive any preventive sexual abuse instruction. Those receiving instruction were more knowledgeable about sexual abuse, more likely to resist attempted abuse, and more likely to report any incidents of abuse that occurred, but they were not any more successful in actually preventing the occurrence of sexual victimization. The telephone survey was repeated 15 months later, which enabled the investigators to study more children who had received a SAP program in the interim and to assess the longer-term effects of those who had received training earlier (Finkelhor, Asdigian, & Dziuba-Leatherman, 1995b). Unfortunately, results of this follow-up replicated the major findings of the initial study.

The Finkelhor et al. (1995a,b) studies are likely to be widely cited and discussed. The data are limited to retrospective self-reports and analyses did not distinguish among different types of victimization (touching, kissing, oral–genital contact, and so on). Furthermore, the quality of sexual instruction provided to respondents could not be judged. Most respondents first learned about sexual abuse through school programs that do not necessarily follow good training practices. Whereas research suggests that multisession, behaviorally oriented approaches are effective in teaching personal safety skills related to sexual abuse, one-shot informational programs predominate in schools (Kohl, 1993). Nevertheless, the Finkelhor et al. (1995a,b) findings give pause with respect to the impact of intervention in preventing sexual assaults.

Several other conclusions have emerged as the SAP research literature has expanded (MacMillan et al., 1994b; Melton, 1992) On the positive side; (1) teachers and parents can be effectively trained to conduct interventions in schools and at home; (2) programs do not appear to make children unduly fearful or anxious, although the possibility of negative side effects should always be assessed; (3) children do not appear to make false reports of abuse following instruction; (4) school programs seem to stimulate parent–child discussions at home about sexual abuse; and (5) training does seem to promote more disclosure of abuse by children and more reporting of suspected abuse by teachers.

There are still several unknowns, however: (1) Does child disclosure of abuse increase support for the child and reduce the trauma of the abuse? (2) How does intervention affect children's later sexual development? and (3) What effects do child-focused interventions have on potential molesters who can be persistent and resourceful in their efforts to victimize children? The latter issue reflects a major limitation in current SAP programs. It seems unlikely that rates of sexual abuse can be substantially reduced without focusing on the factors that prompt adults and older peers to abuse young children. Intervention with potential abusers is quite difficult, however, because there are no good ways to identify those who are at risk to sexually abuse children.

Indicated (Secondary) Prevention

This section discusses indicated prevention for both physical and sexual abuse that involves early intervention after abuse has occurred. This early intervention could provide support for the child during a traumatic period and reduce the likelihood of further abuse, since abuse tends to be repetitive rather than a one-time event. Unfortunately, it is not always possible to determine precisely when behaviors qualify as abusive. Project 12-Ways (Lutzker & Rice, 1987) straddles the fence, so to speak, between primary and secondary prevention. It is a program providing services to parents who have recently been identified by local child protective agencies as having committed abuse and to parents who are considered at high risk for abuse because of the family situation and dynamics. Therefore, some of the target groups have already abused their children, whereas others have not but are at risk to do so.

Project 12-Ways uses behavioral techniques and offers home-based treatment on an individualized basis according to families' needs. Services have included methods to improve home safety, specific training in child management, money management, self-control, and job-finding skills and methods to enhance parents' affectionate behavior toward their children. An evaluation involving 352 families who received services over a 5-year period indicated a 25% reduction in abuse compared to families receiving regular state child protective services. Unfortunately, a later evaluation of Project 12-Ways (Wesch & Lutzker, 1991) indicated that comparable rates of subsequent abuse occurred in treated and comparison families. Analyses suggested, however, that the project sample contained more families with chronic and multiple problems. In other words, Project 12-Ways was successful with more difficult to treat families.

Another approach at secondary prevention is to train physicians, parents, and teachers to identify and report signs of abuse and offer support to children who have been victimized. For instance, school personnel are in a key position to observe signs of both physical and sexual abuse, but in one national survey two thirds of teachers felt that the training they received on maltreatment was insufficient (Abrahams, Casey, & Daro, 1992).

As an example of a teacher training program on sexual abuse, Randolph and Gold (1994) taught teachers how to identify signs of abuse, communicate with children regarding sexual abuse, and how to report suspected cases. Sexual abuse tends to arouse strong emotions in others such as anger, confusion, and sadness. An interesting feature of this training program was the inclusion of exercises designed to help teachers become aware of their own feelings regarding abuse and how to deal with them. Hypothetical vignettes describing sexual abuse were presented to the teachers who were asked to discuss what feelings these situations produced in them. Another exercise was used to develop teachers' empathy for the child. Teachers were asked to pair off with one another and discuss details of their last sexual encounter so they could feel what it was like to disclose intimate information.

Training significantly improved teachers' knowledge about the signs of sexual abuse and increased their inclinations about reporting abuse. Teachers also improved their ability to respond to hypothetical situations related to abuse. A 3-month follow-up indicated several enduring training effects. Teachers reported that they spent significantly more time discussing child abuse with friends or colleagues, led more classroom activities and discussions about abuse, and discussed abuse more frequently with individual children. Finally, trained teachers also reported more instances of suspected abuse to authorities.

In summary, secondary prevention approaches have value in helping families in which abuse has occurred and in prompting the early identification and reporting of abuse. More information is needed, however, to indicate how children are helped by such interventions.

SUMMARY

Although there has not been a great deal of systematic outcome research, there is the suggestion from a few well-conducted programs that it is possible to prevent child physical abuse. Intensive programs begun before the child's birth or very soon after and focused on high-risk populations have shown promise. In terms of sexual abuse, evidence is lacking that teaching children sexual abuse concepts and personal safety skills actually prevents future victimizations, although intervention can improve knowledge and increase the reporting of any abuse that does occur. This is important, since disclosure of sexual abuse is more likely to prevent its repetition and can lead to quick intervention for the child and family.

8

Is Prevention Cost-Effective?

INTRODUCTION

Determining whether programs are worthwhile on a cost basis is an important issue. Resources are limited in all communities and cost analyses can help determine which programs are the best social investments. All program decisions (including decisions not to offer programs) have advantages (benefits) and disadvantages (costs). Cost analyses compare program benefits and costs systematically in an attempt to gain another perspective on the impact of an intervention.

Cost analyses can be very useful from a policy perspective in helping to answer two basic questions: (1) Is society at large (or a particular group) better off with a program than without it? (2) If a program is to be offered, which alternative is best for achieving specific objectives (Barnett & Escobar, 1987)? Good cost analyses also provide information on what specific resources are needed to launch a program, which groups receive which benefits and incur which costs, and, perhaps, how changes could be made to increase a program's value.

Before the results of specific studies are discussed, four points regarding cost analyses should be kept in mind. First, most existing health and social interventions have not been subjected to any cost analysis. Therefore, much more work needs to be done in comparing the costs and effects of all types of programs. Second, there is no standardized procedure for cost analysis. Investigators may consider different costs and benefits, make different assumptions about these parameters, and use different econometric models and analytical procedures. "What is controversial is not whether benefits and costs should be compared, but *what* to count as benefits and costs and *how* to compare them" (Weisbrod, Test, & Stein, 1980, p. 400, italics are the authors). As a result,

143

it is very important to examine the procedures and assumptions that guide any cost analysis. Some analyses may omit important costs or benefits or be too optimistic or pessimistic in their forecasts.

Third, cost analyses are context specific. Results for a program conducted in one setting are best viewed as an estimate of what might be obtained when that same program is transported to another setting. This is because factors affecting the results of cost analysis such as program delivery costs and characteristics of the target population are apt to differ across settings. For instance, the cost of local resources varies across communities (e.g., training and planning time, staff salaries, physical facilities, and how the program will be advertised and integrated with existing service agencies). The target population in the new setting might also differ in terms of the rate at which they accept and complete the program and their risk levels which might affect a program's success rate.

Fourth, money should not be the only criterion when evaluating programs. Some interventions might be very expensive to implement but produce outcomes that are so important and highly valued by citizens that the program will be viewed positively regardless of its costs. Program costs are, at best, only half of the equation and benefits must also be examined.

This chapter summarizes the results of cost analyses of prevention programs and highlights some important issues when considering costs and benefits. Several additional sources providing explanations and details about cost analyses are highly recommended (Gramlich, 1990; Manning, Keeler, Newhouse, Sloss, & Wasserman, 1991; Yates, 1985).

BENEFIT–COST ANALYSES OF PREVENTION

Table 8.1 summarizes the results of several carefully done benefit–cost analyses of prevention programs. In such analyses benefits and costs are translated into monetary figures and presented as a ratio with benefits listed first. A ratio of 2 to 1 (or 2:1, as it frequently appears in publications) would mean that two dollars in benefits are achieved for every dollar spent.

Space does not permit a detailed listing of the costs and benefits for each program included in Table 8.1. While specific items differ, the major costs have been staff salaries and materials. Major benefits have ranged from cost savings from reduced medical costs (Miller & Galbraith, 1995; Windsor et al., 1993), less need for special education services (Barnett, 1993), lower court and police costs (Lipsey, 1984), and

Table 8.1. Results of Cost–Benefit Analyses in Various Areas of Prevention

Study	Area	Benefit–cost ratio	Comment
Barnett (1993)	Early childhood education	8.74 to 1	Actual figures based on 25-year follow-up
Ginsberg & Silverberg (1994)	Legislation requiring bicycle helmets	3.01 to 1	5-year projection
Miller & Galbraith (1995)	Prevention, children 0–4 years	Total: 13 to 1; medical: 0.87 to 1; work: 2.46 to 1; quality of life: 9.42 to 1	Life-time projection
Lipsey (1984)	Delinquency	Range from 0.17 to 8.79	Most projections above 1.0
Olds et al. (1993)	Child health and abuse	At post: 0.72 to 1; 2-year follow-up: 1.06 to 1	Results for low-income participants
Windsor et al. (1993)	Smoking cessation for pregnant women	45.83 to 1	Lifetime projections

lowered welfare payments (Olds, Henderson, Phelps, Kitzman, & Hanks, 1993). Cost analyses can be performed when program participants are followed over time or projected cost analyses can be done if reasonable estimates of program impact are available. In the latter case, authors use available data to project cost savings (i.e., program benefits) into the future. Examples of both types of analyses are presented in Table 8.1.

Benefit–cost analyses of preventive programs have generally been above 1.0, indicating that these interventions yield more benefits than costs. In fact, some ratios are much higher than 1 (8, 13, or almost 46 to 1), indicating the dramatic positive returns that can come from well-executed programs. The findings in Table 8.1 are more impressive when one realizes that current cost analyses have *underestimated* the full value of prevention. All the studies except for Miller and Galbraith (1995) excluded all personal benefits in their economic calculations. That is, the other studies did not take into consideration what personal and social benefits the program produced in participating children and families.

Miller and Galbraith's (1995) figures are quite revealing in terms of the relative importance of personal benefits to a program's "bottom line." Miller and Galbraith (1995) evaluated childhood injury prevention programs conducted by pediatricians (see Chapter 6) and calculated monetary benefits separately for three types of outcomes: (1) savings from medical costs; (2) benefits from increased work the child could eventually perform if not permanently injured or disabled; and (3) personal benefits, which were calculated using a quality of life index that has been used in other studies. The quality of life index placed a dollar value on the child and family's reduced emotional pain and suffering and better overall quality of life due to injury prevention.

The total benefit–cost ratio for injury prevention was very good, 13 to 1, but 72% of the benefits ($9.42 out of $13.00) was derived from the intervention's personal benefits for children and family members. Such data clearly indicate the importance of considering personal benefits when evaluating program impact. At the same time, their study provokes discussion on what is probably the most controversial aspect of cost analysis: how to assess the personal benefits of intervention.

There is no agreement among cost analysts about how to evaluate personal benefits (Drummond, Torrance, & Mason, 1993; Morrow & Bryant, 1995). In benefit–cost analyses there is the need to derive a single cumulative monetary figure for both costs and benefits so the two can be directly compared. It is extremely difficult, if not impossible, however, to portray some types of personal and social outcomes in dollar terms. To deal with this dilemma, those conducting benefit–cost analyses have basically used two approaches. The first, which is more common, includes only results that can be translated easily into monetary terms. The second approach uses one of several different methods such as a quality of life index to capture personal and social benefits (e.g., Miller & Galbraith, 1995). Qualify of life measures transpose outcomes into dollar figures using a willingness to pay strategy. What are individuals willing to pay to live longer, have a higher quality of life, or to be free of physical handicaps and serious burdens?

There are serious limitations with both of the above approaches. The first approach in which the only thing that matters is money clearly biases the evaluation against most social interventions. The major rationale for most preventive programs is to improve the personal and social lives of children and their families. If these outcomes are not considered, then valid conclusions about a program's worth cannot be reached. The second approach is unlikely to capture the true benefits of intervention satisfactorily. It is particularly difficult to quantify the decidedly positive benefits of interventions in economic terms. For instance, how meaningful is it to place a monetary value on the following outcomes: children's enhanced self-esteem, students liking school more, the joy and pleasure of a happy family life, better parenting, a teacher's heightened sense of job satisfaction, or the goodwill and pride created within a community that offers a successful program? While it is technically possible to measure the above outcomes in dollar terms, the final results are likely to be incomplete, unsatisfactory, or misleading. An alternative is cost-effectiveness analysis that can include relevant personal and social benefits. This strategy is discussed later in the chapter.

Several studies in Table 8.1 illustrate other important issues about cost analyses. One study serves as an example that prevention does not have to be highly successful to be cost-effective. Findings from two studies exemplify the need for a long-term perspective in program evaluation. A fourth study is a good example of how different factors interact to influence costs and benefits, and a fifth emphasizes the policy implications of cost analysis. Each of these examples is now briefly discussed.

Example 1: Modest Outcomes Can Be Cost-Effective

The first example involves a smoking cessation program for pregnant women (Windsor et al., 1993); examples of such programs were presented in Chapter 5. Windsor et al. (1993) conducted their study at four maternity clinics serving mostly low-income African-American women and found that a smoking cessation rate of only 14% produced a benefit–cost ratio of 45.83 to 1. Lifetime savings from this smoking cessation program were estimated to be $968,320. These high benefits are possible because of the serious long-term impact of maternal smoking during pregnancy. Based in part on Windsor et al.'s (1993) findings, others have identified smoking cessation programs for pregnant women as one of the most cost-effective interventions available (Tengs et al., 1994).

Examples 2 and 3: Need for Follow-up

Barnett (1985, 1993) has conducted successive evaluations of the Perry Preschool Project (PPP), which was a successful early childhood program designed to prepare high-risk young children for elementary school (see Chapter 3). Because of its intensity, extensiveness, and staffing patterns, PPP was relatively costly to implement. Children participated in PPP for 1 or 2 years when they were 3 or 4 years old, and program costs were $7601 and $14,415, respectively, per child (Barnett, 1993). Although analyses have indicated this initial expense was well worthwhile, it is only because Barnett collected long-term follow-up information that the true value of the program has been revealed.

Approximately 15 years after the preschool program ended, that is, when the children were about 19 years old, the benefit–cost ratios for the 1- and 2-year programs were 1.15 and 0.78, respectively (Barnett, 1985). If the cost analysis of PPP had ended at age 19, the economic return for PPP would be mixed: positive for the 1-year program but slightly negative for the 2-year program. However, follow-up continued for 8 more years and confirmed the cost effectiveness of PPP for *all* participants. A 25-year follow-up reflected positive benefits for children from both the original 1- and 2-year programs. The total net benefit combined across all participating children was *$95,640 per child*. This represents an overall benefit–cost ratio of $8.74 to $1.00 (Barnett, 1993). In other words, every dollar spent on PPP as a preventive preschool intervention eventually returned $8.74 in total benefits. Such data clearly indicate that preventive intervention targeting "human capital" (i.e., the growth and potential of young children) can be a profitable social investment. Such findings should impress decision makers and politicians regardless of their political persuasion.

The importance of follow-up over a much shorter time period is exemplified in the evaluation of a successful home-visiting program described in Chapter 7 that was able to improve a variety of child and maternal health outcomes (Olds et al., 1993). The benefit–cost ratio calculated immediately at the end of the 2½ year program was 0.72, suggesting that the program's benefits had not matched its costs. Two years after the intervention ended, however, the benefit–cost ratio had increased to 1.06, indicating benefits exceeded costs.

The cost analyses conducted by Olds et al. (1993) and Barnett (1985, 1993) confirm the value of adopting a long-term perspective when conducting cost analyses of prevention. If analyses had been restricted to immediate costs and benefits, the net positive value of both interventions would not have been illuminated. Follow-up is important because the costs and benefits of prevention occur at different times. Whereas most costs are incurred when the program is implemented, many benefits might not be apparent until much later when problems do not appear. Because the intent of prevention is to intervene in the present to forestall later problems, it is essential to monitor program participants over sufficiently long enough time periods to assess preventive effects.

Example 4: Factors Interact to Determine Outcomes

Lipsey (1984) conducted a detailed analysis of a delinquency prevention program to illustrate how three important factors interact to influence a program's economic results: (1) the risk status of the partici-

pant; (2) the program's success rate; and (3) different cost-savings projections. The program that was evaluated involved 13 affiliated agencies
in Los Angeles County that offered short-term family counseling and
other services for youth who already had come in contact with the law.
This program is therefore secondary rather than primary prevention,
because treated youth were already showing some behavioral problems.
At the time of intervention, each youth was not at the same level of risk
for subsequent delinquency because of their past behavior, family situation, and so on. For example, within the 70% risk group, seven out of ten
youths are likely to commit delinquent acts in the absence of any intervention. Outcome data from the Los Angeles agencies suggested the
program's success rate in preventing future delinquency ranged between 20 to 40% across the 13 affiliated agencies.

The third factor considered by Lipsey was the estimated cost savings (i.e., benefits) obtainable through intervention. There could be
high, medium, or low cost savings for the local police and courts as well
as savings to victims in terms of personal injury and property damage
and loss depending on the seriousness and repetitive character of the
delinquent acts that are prevented. Table 8.2 contains some of the
benefit–cost ratios calculated by Lipsey (1984) for different risk levels
and success rates and for three cost-savings projections: the least and
most optimistic estimates and an intermediate figure. The benefit–cost
ratios in Table 8.2 indicate that the economic value of delinquency

**Table 8.2. Benefit–Cost Ratios
for Delinquency Prevention as a Function
of Client Risk Level, Treatment Success Rates,
and Cost Savings Projections**

Delinquency risk	Success rate	Cost savings projections		
		Lowest	Intermediate	Highest
15%	20%	0.17	0.30	0.94
	30%	0.26	0.46	1.41
	40%	0.35	0.59	1.88
50%	20%	0.64	1.09	3.45
	30%	0.96	1.63	5.81
	40%	1.28	2.18	6.91
70%	20%	0.81	1.39	4.40
	30%	1.22	2.08	6.59
	40%	1.62	2.77	8.79

Note. Data are drawn from Lipsey (1984). Ratios greater than 1.0 indicate
program benefits exceed costs.

prevention depends on interacting factors. In most scenarios the ratios are above 1.0. In the most positive case (70% risk, a 40% success rate, and the most optimistic cost-saving projection), the program returns $8.79 for every dollar spent. In the worst case (15% risk, 20% success rate, and least optimistic cost saving), the program is not cost-effective (the ratio is 0.17). However, it is encouraging that at the middle levels of each factor (that is, 50% risk, 30% success rate, and and intermediate cost-saving projections), the benefit–cost ratio is 1.63.

Lipsey's (1984) data indicate how different factors interact to influence the results of cost analyses. Furthermore, some factors have stronger implications for program practices than others. Lipsey (1984) noted, for instance, that it was perhaps easier for the Los Angeles program to become more cost-effective by carefully selecting its clients (i.e., by targeting those at higher vs. lower risk for delinquency). Working with certain clients would be easier to do than increasing the success of a treatment to beyond 40% for such a difficult problem like delinquency.

Example 5: Cost Analysis with an Explicit Policy Thrust

Although any cost analysis can be useful in guiding policy deliberations, Ginsberg and Silverberg (1994) conducted a projected benefit–cost analysis that was explicitly done for policy purposes. These authors determined that legislation requiring all bicyclists to wear helmets in Israel would be cost-effective. Helmet legislation would produce a benefit–cost ratio of 3.01 to 1 over a 5-year period and would result in a net savings of $43.3 million and 57 lives to Israeli society. Economic benefits would result even if free bicycle helmets were provided for all potential riders. The authors advocated passage of legislation requiring bicycle helmets because of the savings in money and lives such legislation would probably produce.

COST-EFFECTIVENESS ANALYSIS

In contrast to benefit–cost analysis, the results of a cost-effectiveness analysis are not reduced to a single summary statistic such as a benefit–cost ratio, but involve a detailed listing of different costs and benefits. Some costs and benefits are expressed in monetary terms, some are quantified without estimating their economic value (such as the number of hours required to conduct a program), and the remaining outcomes are described or listed so that they are not overlooked. Cost-effectiveness analyses can accommodate more of the personal benefits of intervention, especially those that are difficult if not impossible to translate into dollar figures. Therefore, cost-effectiveness analyses are generally preferred when evaluating prevention programs.

One way to handle outcomes that cannot be translated into monetary figures is to present the results of cost-effectiveness analyses in other ways. Alternative programs can be compared in terms of their relative costs to achieve the same valued nonmonetary outcome. For instance, analyses can show that it costs one program $500.00 per student to raise reading achievement scores of high-risk children to grade level; it may cost another program only $300.00 to achieve the same result. Or, in another way to illustrate results, program A may cost $450.00 to prevent the future onset of each incident of clinical depression, whereas program B can attain the same result for $200.00.[1] These types of comparisons can help determine which intervention is preferred in achieving the same goals.

Although there have not yet been any detailed cost-effectiveness analyses of prevention programs, Table 8.3 provides a guide for such analyses. The hypothetical intervention relevant to Table 8.3 is a school-based effort by teachers to prevent academic and behavioral problems in elementary schoolchildren. The program also includes evening sessions for parents to improve their child-rearing skills. Inspection of Table 8.3 indicates that potentially relevant program costs and benefits fall into eight categories. There are two cost categories (direct and indirect costs) and six benefit categories that assess direct or indirect benefits to children, families, schools, and society. Some of these categories are now briefly discussed.

Time as a Program Cost

Most of the program costs listed in Table 8.3 are relatively straightforward, but one frequently overlooked cost is time, which is a valuable commodity. There is no such thing as "free" time. Citizens may choose not to participate in programs because they feel they have more valuable ways to spend their time. Time commitments can also be critical when choosing among program alternatives.

For example, King (1994) compared the costs of three academic programs in terms of the financial expenses involved and the amount of time required of teachers, principals, and parents to conduct the program. The most expensive program from a financial standpoint was the least expensive in terms of time requirements. From a policy or adop-

[1] I am indebted to Amiram Vinokur for bringing this issue to my attention.

Table 8.3. Possible Costs and Benefits for a Cost-Effectiveness Analysis

Hypothetical program: A school-based intervention implemented by teachers that contains separate classroom components designed to improve children's academic functioning and their social skills. Biweekly evening meetings at the school to enhance parental child-rearing skills are also part of the program.

Possible Program Costs

I. Direct costs
    1. Initial training of teachers and other school staff
    2. Ongoing supervision, consultation, and staff development
    3. Salaries of any additional staff required (e.g., to work with parents)
    4. Supplies and materials
    5. Use of facilities (school space for parent meetings)
    6. Program evaluation costs
    7. Negative side effects occurring in:
        a. School staff
        b. Parents or siblings
        c. Child participants
    8. Time required of:
        a. Teachers, principals, and other school staff
        b. Parents
        c. Students
II. Indirect costs
    1. Parent transportation to meetings
    2. Child care (for parents to attend meetings)
    3. Alterations in existing school curriculum to accommodate the new program (must something be dropped?)

Possible Program Benefits

III. Direct benefits due to reduction in child problems
    1. Less need of special education services
    2. Less need of school-based mental health services
    3. Lower rate of grade retention
    4. Reduced stress, symptomatology among children
    5. Reduced social dysfunction (less peer rejection)
IV. Direct benefits to children due to increased competencies
    1. Improved social skills
    2. Improved academic functioning
    3. Enhanced psychological well-being (e.g., self-efficacy, happiness)
V. Direct benefits to other participants
    1. Gains in self-efficacy, self-confidence in
        a. Teachers
        b. Parents
    2. Positive effects on siblings
    3. Enhanced family functioning
    4. Teachers' increased job satisfaction
    5. Increased social support for/among school staff

Table 8.3. (*Continued*)

　　6.　Lower stress, anxiety, or burden in
　　　a.　Parents
　　　b.　Teachers
　　　c.　Siblings
VI.　Possible indirect benefits for all participants
　　1.　Children's enhanced social relationships (with peers, teachers, family members)
　　2.　Improved school climate or atmosphere
　　3.　Improved teacher–parent relationships
　　4.　Improved image/reputation of school in local media and community
　　5.　Reduced need for health care and mental health treatment in the community for children or family members
　　6.　Less need for community-based social and criminal justice services
　　7.　Heightened community goodwill and sense of pride in offering a successful program
VII.　Other possible benefits
　　1.　External benefits due to reductions in external costs
　　2.　Greater educational attainment for children
　　3.　Greater vocational attainment for children
　　4.　Children participate in and contribute more positively to society.
　　5.　Increased tax revenues (children ultimately go farther in school and gain higher-paying jobs)
VIII.　Practical benefits: Consumer reactions to the intervention
　　1.　What proportion of the eligible or target population participated?
　　2.　What proportion completed the program?
　　3.　How acceptable were program practices to consumers?
　　4.　How satisfied were program participants with obtained outcomes?

Note. Attempts should be made to determine how different stakeholders, including subgroups of participants, incur different costs and derive different benefits.

tion perspective, then, the choice among programs would best be made according to available resources. For schools who have the financial resources but who cannot gain sufficient time commitments from relevant groups, one program would be the best choice, while another program would be preferable for schools in opposite circumstances. Unless the different costs required to implement a program are clearly specified, however, one cannot make the best informed choice about what program is most appropriate for a particular setting. King's (1994) analysis also suggests that a program's nonmonetary costs (in this case, time) can be just as important as its monetary expenditures.

Program Benefits

　　As Table 8.3 suggests, there are different benefits derived from reducing problems and from promoting health that should be considered (see Table 8.3, sections III to VII). In the former case, children can benefit because their stress and anxiety is reduced, they are not being rejected or taunted by peers, their parents and teachers are less punitive, or they experience less difficulty in learning. In terms of health promotion, children can also benefit because they become happier and more self-confident, earn better grades, like school more, or gain friends who are supportive. In a corresponding fashion, parents or teachers may benefit from either reduced stress and burden or increased role satisfaction and self-confidence. Note, however, how difficult it would be to translate the above benefits into dollar figures.

Stakeholder Perspectives

As suggested in Table 8.3, a program is likely to affect teachers, parents, and participating children and society in general in different ways. It is very important to understand how benefits and costs vary across groups. Cost analysts refer to this as assessing the equity or distributional effects of interventions and often consider the perspectives of at least four groups of stakeholders: program participants (including their family member), nonparticipants (usually identified as taxpayers), agency sponsors, and society as a whole. Cost and benefits are rarely shared equally by different stakeholders.

For instance, some subgroups of participants may benefit more than others. The program may work more effectively for members of high socioeconomic groups, for males, for younger children, or for families of certain ethnic or cultural backgrounds. Having this information is extremely important because some programs may have to be modified to increase benefits for certain groups.

Stakeholders also bear different costs of the intervention. For instance, in the hypothetical example, teachers have the added responsibility of learning a new intervention; they must devote their time and energy to this task and then incorporate the program into their customary routine and perhaps make some adjustments to the operation of their classrooms. These personal costs are not borne by other stakeholders.

Agencies also differ in sharing program benefits and costs. Some agencies must pay for the initial costs of the program while it is being implemented, while others reap the program's major benefits in the future. For example, an elementary school that pays in terms of money, staff, and resources for a successful intensive intervention for all of its first graders would see some benefits, but middle, junior, and senior high schools are in the most preferential position. These latter schools would reap the rewards of having better functioning and achieving students without having to pay for the initial program. Politicians and administrators often have a very time-limited perspective and focus on yearly budgets; it may be difficult to convince them to fund prevention programs now that will save money and produce benefits several years later. In some cases, however, taxpayers may be more willing to vote for higher school taxes or fund other community projects if the data from cost analyses indicate how they and their community profit from prevention programs.

Importance of External Benefits

In Table 8.3, section VII, external benefits are mentioned. These benefits are frequently overlooked and deserve some extended discussion. External benefits are those that occur for society at large or for taxpayers. External benefits result when the frequently hidden or overlooked external costs of problems are eliminated or reduced.

For example, Manning et al. (1991) have indicated that there are substantial external costs associated with three unhealthy habits: smoking, drinking, and not exercising. External costs connected with these habits consist of such things as collectively financed group health, life, and disability insurance plans, retirement pensions, lifetime taxes on earnings, and, depending on the habit, items such as the effect of passive smoking on others. In many public and private employee benefit plans all workers and employers pay the same premiums regardless of their health habits. Basically, this mean that nonsmokers are subsidizing smokers, nondrinkers are subsidizing drinkers, and so on. At the same time, smokers and heavy drinkers have shorter life expectancies and thus shorter working lives and will pay less in taxes to support governmental programs.

Manning et al. (1991) emphasized that each of the three unhealthy habits they studied was costly to society and that heavy drinking (defined as five or more drinks per day) was the most costly. On a per capita basis, total lifetime external costs were estimated at $1000 for each smoker, $1650 per sedentary (nonexercising) person, and $42,000 for each heavy drinker. The greater costs for drinking are derived primarily from the loss of innocent lives and property damage due to vehicle accidents and the additional social and medical services that must be expended to address the problems of heavy drinkers.

Programs that prevent unhealthy habits thus turn external costs that would otherwise be imposed on society into external benefits. Including external benefits in a cost analysis can greatly enhance the perceived value of prevention. For example, an intervention that prevents only ten adolescents from drinking heavily yields lifetime external benefits to society of $420,000. Cost analyses of prevention program should somehow try to evaluate any external benefits that occur, since such benefits probably exist for all problems that can be prevented such as unintentional injury, poor school achievement, and various behavioral problems.

Consumer Reactions

Finally, one should not overlook consumer reactions to intervention (Table 8.3, section VIII). It is helpful to gather data on what proportion of the eligible population elects to participate, if they perceive program practices to be suitable and acceptable to their lifestyle, how many complete the program, and if they are satisfied with the outcomes they achieve. Consumer reactions can be an important indicator of how well a program is attentive to local needs and preferences. Wolf (1978) offers a good discussion of the importance of assessing consumer reactions to interventions.

Comparing Alternative Interventions

As more cost analyses of health and social interventions are reported, it will become possible to compare different policies and programs. Given a choice between two programs, which is the better alternative? Such comparisons will probably confirm the wisdom of the saying, "You get what you pay for." Some programs may not cost much, but they produce so little benefit that they are not really a bargain. This is the case with brief informational programs that rarely produce any significant behavioral change. Other programs may be relatively more costly but preferable because they produce substantially better outcomes.

Furthermore, even if evaluations suggest prevention is costly in a particular circumstance, prevention can still be a better option in the long run than treating those who later develop problems. For example, in light of the very high social and personal costs associated with alcohol and drug abuse, it has been estimated that on a nationwide basis, drug abuse prevention has a benefit–cost ratio of $14.89 to $1 (Kim, Williams, Coletti, Hepler, & Crutchfield, 1995). Although this is a crude estimate drawn from national data on rates and costs of drug abuse, it suggests the possible value of prevention over treatment. Several other difficult to treat problems come to mind that have serious and costly long-term consequences: externalizing problems, academic difficulties, teenage pregnancy, and many health problems such as serious birth defects, obesity, and coronary heart disease. For instance, in 1980, 41% of all medical expenditures in the United States went to serving 17% of the population who had one or more chronic disabling conditions (Rice & LaPlante, 1992). Prevention does not necessarily have to be highly successful in the above situations to be a better social investment than treatment. Prevention might not always be less expensive than treatment (Russell, 1986), but, once again, money should not be the only consideration.

A Caution

I want to return to comments offered at the beginning of this chapter that cost analyses are *one* way to determine the value of social interventions, but certainly not the only way. Although current cost analyses of prevention have been favorable, promoting prevention because of its potential cost-effectiveness has at least three risks. One, politicians, administrators, and funding agencies may focus on costs rather than benefits and claim that a complete program cannot be afforded at this time, but a more modest one can be supported. It can be a mistake, however, to offer "watered-down" programs; that is, to replicate some of the exemplary programs described in this book in a very limited way in order to save money. Prevention should not be attempted "on the cheap," so to speak. The critical features of many successful programs are unknown, and reducing the length and intensity of intervention, asking staff to serve greatly expanded numbers of clients, and using other means of cutting corners to save expenses could totally undermine a program's impact. Rogers, Peoples-Sheps, and Sorenson (1995) offer an example of what can happen.

Two, promoting prevention solely because of its cost-effectiveness may play into the hands of those who would argue that data from such analyses must be available before prevention can be actively promoted. Frank (1993) has noted that in the past such arguments have often been politically motivated and were used to reduce budgets for innovative programs or to avoid paying for new programs. The argument of requesting more information on cost-effectiveness before doing more prevention imposes a higher standard on prevention programs than therapy, rehabilitation, or remedial interventions whose current existence is almost never justified on the basis of cost-effectiveness.

Three, a favorable cost analysis does not inevitably lead to the adoption of more prevention programs or the rejection of existing programs. For example, Frank (1993) cited examples of mental health programs that were found to be very cost-effective compared to existing treatments, but were nevertheless not adopted by existing service providers. Therefore, the fact that a program is cost-effective in no way guarantees its acceptance or adoption by others.

In summary, although cost analyses are helpful, a primary focus should be on program quality: How is the program working and who is being well served? When the priority becomes improving program quality instead of cutting costs, then attention is appropriately directed at meeting the needs of the community rather than the program's economic bottom line.

SUMMARY

A cost analysis comparing the benefits and costs of an intervention is one useful criterion that can be used in evaluating the value of any program, although it should not be the only one. Cost analyses should be as comprehensive as possible to provide an accurate picture of a program's worth. This means two things: (1) that all relevant costs and benefits are considered, and (2) participants are followed for a sufficiently long enough period to assess preventive effects. Although only a few cost evaluations of prevention programs have been reported, their results suggest that prevention is a worthwhile social investment. The ratio of benefits over costs has generally been greater than one, and in some cases, prevention has returned over $8, $13, or $45 in benefits for every dollar spent. Furthermore, most current benefit–cost analyses have underestimated the full value of prevention by insufficiently considering and evaluating personal benefits. Compared to benefit–cost analyses, cost-effectiveness analyses list and describe any costs and benefits that cannot be easily translated into monetary terms. Cost-effectiveness analyses can also compare programs in terms of their relative costs in achieving valued nonmonetary outcomes. As a result, cost-effectiveness analysis can provide a more complete picture of program impact, and thus be more appropriate for prevention.

9

Importance of Policy

INTRODUCTION

In general, social policy refers to the rules governing the behavior of individuals in a particular setting. Sometimes, the rules are fixed such as in regulations or laws; at other times, the rules are more flexible such as a policy that authorizes new services but does not specify exactly service delivery or eligibility. At a very fundamental level, social policies serve as guidelines in managing relationships and distributing available resources among individuals, groups, institutions, and communities.

The preventive implications of social policy are often overlooked, although effective policies can influence behavior in several ways (McLeroy, Bibeau, Steckler, & Glantz, 1988). Policies can reduce unwanted behaviors in settings (via no-smoking bans) or for certain age groups (by establishing minimal ages for purchasing and consuming alcohol and tobacco products). Policies can decrease behavior by increasing its costs (via taxation) and increase or decrease access to services (by eliminating barriers or establishing eligibility requirements). Most importantly, by creating structures that provide administrative support and funding for programs, policies can strongly influence the types and duration of research and service. Therefore, social policy initiatives can play an important role in a total public health effort at prevention.

Several interventions involving policy matters have been discussed in previous chapters relating to the prevention of behavioral and academic problems and drug use (see Chapters 2–4). The current chapter focuses on additional policy initiatives, particularly the use of laws and

taxation affecting drug use, and is intended as a general introduction to
the importance of a policy perspective. Several other sources provide
excellent theoretical and practical discussions of issues related to mental health (Mechanic, 1989), physical health (Kronenfeld, 1993), and
family policies (Zimmerman, 1995).

Overview of Policy Research

Research indicates that factors related to the content, implementation, and ecological fit of a policy affect its ultimate impact (Palumbo &
Calista, 1990). A policy should be drafted so that its elements are appropriate for the target population and behavior(s) in question; the policy
must also be realistic and attainable and as comprehensive and consistent as possible. Then the policy must be correctly implemented, which
means securing sufficient resources for its enactment or enforcement.
Finally, a policy must be consistent with the values and norms of a
setting and population or the policy will probably be ignored or undermined in some way. If matters relating to policy content, implementation, and fit are not handled effectively, then the resultant policy is
much less likely to have its intended effect. Examples are provided in
the following sections of this chapter.

EFFECTS OF SPECIFIC POLICIES

School Policies

Data from one research group underscore the importance of consistency and comprehensiveness in school policies. Pentz et al. (1989)
assessed four components of schools' smoking policies: (1) if the smoking policy was written and regularly enforced; (2) if there was a closed
campus (so students could not leave the school grounds and smoke
during the day); (3) if smoking was restricted near school grounds; and
(4) if smoking prevention was part of the school curricula. There was a
significant negative relationship between the number of policy components in place and the level of student smoking in 23 middle and junior
high California schools. For example, students in schools whose policies contained all four components showed 38% less smoking than
those in schools with only two components.

If consistency and comprehensiveness are important, then many
changes should be made in existing school policies. One survey of over
200 schools found that although all schools had some form of smoking

policy, many children nevertheless received inconsistent or contradictory messages about smoking (Bowen, Kinne, & Orlandi, 1995). In 10% of elementary schools and 26% of high schools, smoking was not allowed during the school day but was permitted at events occurring after school hours such as sports and music events. Only 29% of elementary schools and 50% of high schools were totally smoke-free (banned employee as well as student smoking). The school's smoking policies were publicly displayed in only half of the schools. Finally, many school curricula either paid token attention to smoking or relied on informational approaches, which are now known to be ineffective.

Another survey of a nationally representative sample of private and public schools examined school policies regarding drugs, smoking, and violence (Ross et al., 1995). Several limitations in school policies were noted. For instance, 23 to 50% of schools did not explicitly define the behavior the policy was intended to affect (what does violence entail?); 26 to 44% did not have any procedure in place for communicating their policy to students, staff, and parents; 40 to 58% lacked specific procedures to implement the relevant policy; and, finally, 28 to 78% did not make any specific efforts at preventive education. In each case, the lower percentages noted above refer to policies regarding drug use and the higher numbers refer to policies involving tobacco or violence. Therefore, policies in many local schools must be improved if they are to have their intended effect.

Taxation of Tobacco Products

Taxation is one type of social policy that can be used to influence drug use based on the basic economic principle that there is a negative relationship between price and demand. Most experts agree that raising the price of cigarettes and alcoholic beverages does lower the purchase and consumption of these products by young people (Manning, Blumberg, & Moulton, 1995; Peterson, Zeger, Remington, & Anderson, 1992). Hence, cigarette smoking and alcohol use can be reduced among young people (although not completely eliminated) by increasing product prices through taxation. For example, there was a substantial drop in national sales of cigarettes in the United State following the doubling of the federal excise tax on cigarettes in January 1983 from 8 to 16 cents per pack (Peterson et al., 1992). Evaluating the data on a state-by-state basis from 1955 to 1988, Peterson et al. (1992) reported that a clear relationship between state taxation and cigarette consumption also emerged: Consumption declined in states that increased taxes and rose over time in states without tax increases.

Another example of the influence of taxes comes from a study evaluating the relative effects of taxation and an antismoking media campaign in California (Hu, Sung, & Keeler, 1995). In 1988, the state of California increased state cigarette taxes by 250%, from 10 to 35 cents per pack, and used part of the revenues to fund a subsequent statewide antismoking media campaign. Because the media campaign followed the tax increase, it was possible to compare their relative effects. The state tax was over three times more effective in reducing cigarette consumption than the media campaign, although both interventions had positive effects. Over a 30-month period, the tax led to a 9.5% reduction in cigarette smoking, whereas the media campaign reduced smoking by an additional 2.7%.[1]

Taxation of tobacco products is very low in the United States compared to Canada, which has imposed substantial taxes on cigarettes since 1981. In 1991, tobacco taxes averaged only 38 cents in the United States, accounting for approximately 20% of the cost of a package of cigarettes. In contrast, Canadian taxes were *$3.24 per pack*, representing 75% of the retail price (Kaiserman & Rogers, 1991). Along with other public policies, the heavy Canadian taxes on cigarettes are believed to be responsible for reducing adolescent smoking in Canada by up to 62% (Elders et al., 1994).

Taxation of Alcoholic Products

There have only been two federal excise tax hikes on alcoholic beverages (beer, wine, or distilled spirits) since 1951 in the United States. In fact, the real price of alcoholic beverages (i.e., discounted for inflation) is approximately 26% *lower* today than it was in 1975 (Grossman, Chaloupka, Saffer, & Laixuthai, 1994). Unwittingly, the relatively low price for alcoholic beverages is, in effect, a de facto public policy in the United States that *encourages rather than discourages* alcoholic use.

Examining data from several previous nationwide studies, Grossman et al. (1994) confirmed that a significant negative relationship exists between the price and the consumption of alcohol by adolescents. Higher prices are associated with reduced adolescent drinking. Further-

[1]The media campaign may have been more successful than this study indicated. On June 28, 1996, an ABC news documentary, "Never say die: How the cigarette companies keep on winning," reported that an intense lobbying campaign initiated by the tobacco industry was successful in diverting most of the California tobacco tax money away from the antismoking media campaign. The cigarette companies apparently viewed the media campaign as developing progressively more effective antismoking messages. After the diversion of tax monies, rates of smoking among Californians began to slowly rise.

more, they conducted several mathematical simulations to illustrate the powerful impact of price on consumption. These simulations illustrated how a policy of indexing the federal excise tax on alcohol to the rate of inflation since 1951 coupled with a minimum drinking age of 21 (see discussion below) could have produced strong effects on adolescent drinking. For instance, the percentage of high school seniors who drink frequently could have been reduced by 43%, the percentage reporting at least one heavy drinking episode in the previous 2 weeks could be reduced by 18%, and the percentage of youth abstaining completely from alcohol in the past year could increase by 80%.

Policies relating to alcohol can have the dual effect of reducing drinking and serious injuries among youth. Traffic accidents cause approximately half of all deaths and spinal cord injuries among persons 15 to 19, and alcohol is a contributory factor in a majority of these incidents (Vegega & Klitzner, 1988). An estimated 1000 young lives could be saved each year by increased prices on alcohol, particularly beer, which is the predominant drink of young people. Grossman et al. (1994) conclude: "... if reductions in youth alcohol consumption, heavy alcohol consumption, and alcohol-related injuries and deaths are desired, an increase in federal taxes on alcoholic beverages is an effective policy to accomplish these goals" (p. 362).

Effects of Legislation

Laws are often appealing to the general public and government officials as a quick-fix approach, as though the mere passage of a law will solve a social problem or crisis. Laws should not be seen as a panacea for any social problem, and in some case laws have had virtually no effect. Making drugs such as heroin, marijuana, and cocaine illegal has not been very helpful in reducing the use of such substances. Nevertheless, certain types of legislation, when appropriately crafted and sufficiently implemented, can have a positive impact and become part of an overall public health approach in prevention. The following sections first discuss no-smoking laws and then the impact of laws related to alcohol.

Clean Air Laws

The number of clean air (no-smoking) laws increased tenfold in the United States between 1980 and 1989, and by July 1989, 44 states and over 500 cities had adopted this type of legislation in some form (Rigotti & Pashos, 1991). Clean air laws are usually passed to reduce secondhand smoke exposure for nonsmokers, but they can have the dual effect of preventing smoking. For instance, there are data to support the notion that making it more difficult to smoke can reduce the number of young people who will take up the habit in the first place.

Using data drawn from across the United States, Wasserman, Manning, Newhouse, and Winkler (1991) reported that there was a significant negative relationship between the presence of clean air laws and smoking behavior for both adults and adolescents, but that adolescents appear to be more strongly affected by such legislation. In fact, they estimated that if no-smoking laws were extended to the maximum number of sites possible (i.e., government buildings, restaurants, public transportation, recreational and cultural events, schools, and so on), adolescent smoking could be reduced by 41%. Furthermore, analyses suggested that clean air laws had a relatively stronger impact on teenagers' decisions to begin smoking compared to reducing cigarette consumption among current smokers. Therefore, it does seem that no-smoking laws can be one effective component of a public policy approach regarding smoking.

Drunk-Driving Laws

Determining the effects of various laws deterring alcohol use (so-called drunk-driving laws) is complicated (Chaloupka, Saffer, & Grossman, 1993; Grossman et al., 1994; Snortum, 1988). First, drunk-driving laws vary substantially across the United States and include different combinations of statutes related to mandatory breath testing, levels of blood alcohol that determine drunkenness, server liability laws, and specific penalties such as loss of license, fines, community service, or jail terms. Moreover, some penalties are automatic, while others escalate in severity based on successive convictions. In addition to this plethora of regulations, there are many other factors that influence adolescent drinking such as adult and peer use of alcohol, religiosity, sex and race, public opinion, media coverage, bureaucratic commitment, and social norms.

Second, compliance with any legislation that is essentially punitive in nature such as drunk-driving laws depends heavily on citizens' perceptions of the probability of arrest and the certainty of a penalty (Snortum, 1988; Wagenaar & Wolfson, 1995). This merely illustrates the importance of behavioral consequences. If young people believe that they can effectively evade the law and its consequences, legislation will have little behavioral effect. Unfortunately, vigorous enforcement of drunk-driving laws does not usually occur. In fact, it has been estimated that only 2 out of every 2000 youthful violators of drunk-driving laws are ever arrested (Wolfson, Wagenaar, & Hornseth, 1995). This reality is, of course, not emphasized in community education programs, since the aim of such programs is to convince citizens that if you drive while drunk, you will be caught and you will be punished. Therefore, highly visible efforts by local police and the courts to enforce drunk-driving laws are important. The types of drunk-driving legislation that do seem to reduce the level of drinking and driving among young people are discussed in the following two sections.

Minimum Age Laws.   The clearest evidence that legislation related to alcohol can have a preventive effect involves laws defining the minimum legal age for drinking. O'Malley and Wagenaar (1991) took advantage of changes occurring in minimum drinking age laws in the United States to study the effects of these laws on drinking and fatal vehicle accidents. Whereas in the early 1970s, many states had lowered the minimum drinking age from 21 to 18, 19, or 20, some states maintained their higher legal drinking ages. In response to a federal law passed in 1984, linking states' receipt of highway funds to passage of a minimum drinking age of 21, however, almost all states with lower age limits passed new legislation to once again increase the legal age to 21. Figure 9.1 presents data on alcohol consumption by high school seniors in states that always had a minimum drinking age of 21 (Always-21 States) and in states that initially had a lower drinking age that was later changed to age 21 after 1984 (Change to 21 States). Alcohol consumption was assessed in terms of the frequency of drinking by high school seniors in the past month, and statistical adjustments were made for the typical underreporting of such behaviors.

The data in Fig. 9.1 are presented over 3-year periods and suggest that a higher legal drinking age does affect behavior. This is reflected in three different ways. First, before the federal law was passed in 1984, there were significant differences in the use of alcohol by youth in states with different minimum age laws. High school seniors in the Always-21 states drank significantly less frequently than those in states with lower minimum ages. Second, there was a significant reduction over time in alcohol consumption by students within states that increased their minimum age to 21 after 1984. Third, during the years 1985–1987, when states had similar minimum drinking ages, there were no longer any significant between-state differences in youth's rates of drinking.

What do these data mean in practical terms? Analyses of drinking patterns before 1984 indicated that the prevalence rate for any drinking at all was 5.6% less in states where the legal age was 21 than in other states, and there was a corresponding 2.8% lower rate of heavy drink-

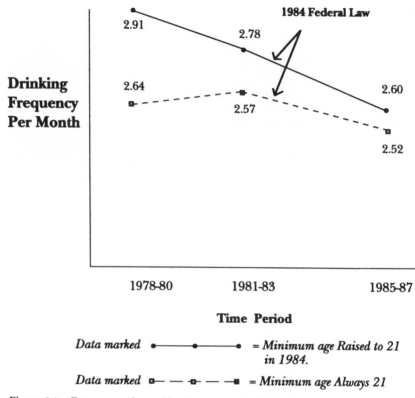

Drinking Frequency Per Month

2.91

2.78

1984 Federal Law

2.64

2.57

2.60

2.52

1978-80   1981-83   1985-87

Time Period

Data marked •————• = *Minimum age Raised to 21 in 1984.*

Data marked ▫— — ▫— — ▪ = *Minimum age Always 21*

Figure 9.1. Frequency of monthly alcohol use by high school seniors in states with different minimum drinking ages before and after the 1984 law linked federal highway funds to a legal minimum age of 21. Data are from O'Malley and Wagenaar (1991).

ing (defined as consuming five or more drinks on any one occasion). Although such differences might seem minor, when projected on a national scale, they are not. In a population of approximately 9 million adolescents aged 17 to 19, if all states had a minimum drinking age of 21, then over one half million fewer youth would have been drinking at all, and 250,000 fewer would have drunk heavily.

Minimum age laws have also saved lives. In states in which the drinking age was increased from 18 to 21, there was a subsequent decline of 26.3% in the rate of fatalities resulting from motor vehicle accidents. Increasing the minimum drinking age to 19 or 20 resulted in a lower but nevertheless substantial decline in fatalities (18.6 and 21.6%, respectively). Moreover, the decline in traffic fatalities occurred only for the under-21 age group, suggesting the specific impact of the law on young people's driving fatalities.

If some data indicate that increasing the driving age saves lives, then one would also expect a reverse effect: Reducing the legal drinking age should cost lives. This is precisely what was reported in a study comparing fatality rates over time in two states and one Canadian province that lowered the drinking age from 21 to 18 in the early 1970s (Williams, Rich, Zador, & Robertson, 1975). Reducing the minimum drinking age was associated with a significant increase in motor vehicle fatalities for drivers under age 21; no change occurred in three contiguous locales that did not change their legal drinking age. In the year following the new legislation, Williams et al. (1975) estimated that 70 youth died in fatal crashes who would have lived if the legal drinking age had been maintained at 21.

Comparing Types of Legislation. Chaloupka et al. (1993) conducted simulation analyses to compare the effects of various types of drunk-driving statutes as well as taxing policies on motor vehicle fatalities among 18 to 20 year olds. Their data confirmed the findings of other researchers that taxation and having a legal minimum age of 21 significantly reduces motor vehicle fatalities among young people; however, other types of legislation also had some effects. For example, a mandatory loss of a driver's license for 1 year after the first offense could reduce traffic fatalities by about 9%. The automatic penalty must be 1 year, however; less severe penalties would have little effect. According to Chaloupka et al. (1993), mandatory breath testing, server liability laws (i.e., holding those who serve alcohol to underage youth liable for damages), and a mandatory fine of $500 for the first offense could also each reduce vehicle deaths by about 5%. Other types of drunk-driving legislation (such as jail sentences and community service) did not seem to deter drunk driving. Although the simulations conducted by Chaploupka et al. (1993) yield estimated effects, their findings can help those attempting to reach decisions on the relative merits of different types of drunk-driving laws.

Limiting Minors' Access to Cigarettes and Alcohol

Sometimes it is the implementation of a policy rather than the policy itself that needs attention. This is illustrated in the next section, which discusses limiting minors' access to tobacco and alcoholic products.

Enforcing Laws Banning Sales to Minors

Although it is illegal to sell cigarettes to those under 18 in almost all states, many commercial retailers (between 34 and 91%, depending on the community) do not comply with the law. "Nearly all adolescent smokers report that they have purchased a pack of cigarettes at least once; a majority of adolescents smokers find the purchase of cigarettes fairly easy" (Elders et al., 1994). As a result, laws designed to reduce smoking among teens by outlawing the sale of tobacco products to minors do not have their intended impact. Retailers' compliance with cigarette sales laws are rarely enforced. One survey in 1989 found that only five states recorded any violations of such laws, and there were only 32 total violations recorded in these states during the entire year (Office of the Inspector General, 1990).

A few studies have sought to influence retailers' compliance with cigarette sales laws either by educational approaches or by encouraging local police to enforce the law. It should come as no surprise that education by itself does not produce much change; enforcement efforts, however, do change retailers' selling practices.

For instance, a merchant education approach by itself was not effective in reducing sales of cigarettes to minors in Erie County, New York (Skretny, Cummings, Sciandra, & Marshall, 1990). Informational packets were sent to randomly selected local businesses. The packets included clear explanations of the relevant ordinance regarding sales to minors, warning signs which by law were to be posted in each establishment, and a tip sheet about how to handle minors who attempted to purchase cigarettes. The educational intervention had little effect. Teenagers who were research confederates were able to purchase cigarettes in 77% of the stores receiving the informational packets and 86% of nonintervention stores. Warning signs were on display in only 40% of the intervention stores.

Another study combined education and enforcement in a single suburban community that had recently passed legislation prohibiting cigarette sales to minors (Jason, Ji, Anes, & Birkhead, 1991). The educational component was comprehensive and targeted schoolchildren, merchants, and all community residents. Merchant education was accomplished by personally visiting each business with a license to sell cigarettes in the community. Local media also publicized this law. Information about the law and requests for compliance were sent to all families with children in the local schools. In the enforcement component of the program, local police conducted quarterly "sting operations" to monitor merchant adherence to the new law by sending underage customers into stores to buy cigarettes.

The combined communitywide effort was successful. Initially, 70% of all stores sold cigarettes to minors as determined by sales to teenage confederates. After the first two quarterly enforcement periods, this rate was cut in half to 35%, and 16 months later only 3% of the stores (actually only one store in the community) sold cigarettes to underage customers.

A final study in California clarified the differential value of education and enforcement by introducing these components successively over time and assessing their effects (Feighery, Altman, & Shaffer, 1991). Four suburban communities were studied. First, a community and merchant education approach was conducted over an initial 4-month period. Information packets were mailed to local merchants explaining California law and its penalties and local media also presented stories about how easy and illegal it was for minors to purchase cigarettes in their community. Second, over the next 4-month period, police sting operations were conducted on a randomly selected group of merchants and citations were issued if stores made illegal sales.

Figure 9.2 presents the results of this intervention. Initially, 72% of all stores sold tobacco to minors over the counter; this number dropped slightly to 62% after the educational intervention, but it fell more dramatically to 21% following police enforcement. In other words, adding police enforcement to the community education approach was much more effective than the educational approach alone in reducing illegal cigarette sales.

Whereas the above studies focused on sales of cigarettes to minors, the situation is similar for alcohol. Alcohol is easily obtainable by underage youth and law enforcement is generally lax. In one 3-year period, more than 25% of 295 counties took no administrative actions against retailers for selling alcohol to minors (Wagenaar & Wolfson, 1995). There also seemed to be a misplaced emphasis when enforcement did occur. The typical county was 17 times more likely to direct penalties at the underage youth than the commercial establishment providing the alcohol. Yet, data indicate that enforcement directed at alcohol retailers does have an effect. Preusser and Williams (1992) found that underage consumers could purchase alcoholic beverages from local vendors 80% of the time in Westchester county, New York, and 97% of the time in the Washington, DC, area, but only 35% of the time in Albany county, New York, where local police periodically enforce minimum

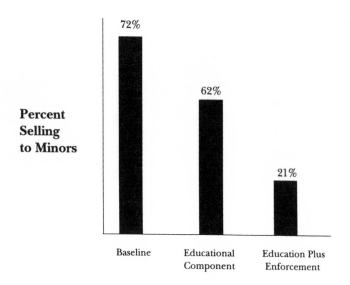

72%

62%

**Percent
Selling
to Minors**

21%

Baseline   Educational   Education Plus
                Component   Enforcement

Phase of Intervention

Figure 9.2. Percentage of retailers selling cigarettes to minors over the counter during different phases of an intervention. Data are from Feighery, Altman, and Shaffer (1991).

age drinking laws by conducting sting operations and fining merchants who sell to underage customers.

Barriers to Enforcement

Police may be reluctant to enforce some types of legislation for a variety of reasons: because administrative support is lacking, other aspects of their job seem more important, or due to a personal reluctance to punish someone who has not violated any other law. For instance, one group of investigators found that police were very reluctant to enforce a new child safety seat law (Lavelle, Hovell, West, & Walgren, 1992). Police believed that fining drivers $50.00 for lack of a child safety seat (as indicated by the law) was too aversive a procedure. Because it appeared unlikely that police would enforce the law as prescribed, a compromise was struck. Instead of the customary $50 fine, a referral coupon was issued to each noncompliant driver. The coupon entitled drivers to have the $50 fine waived if they attended an educational workshop and purchased a child safety seat. A series of nine training sessions for police was held that explained this coupon system, the enforcement procedures for the new law, and the rationale for the legislation in terms of how it was expected to save young children's lives.

Data were collected over a 4.5-year period, including before the car seat law was enacted, following its enactment and police enforcement training, and over a 6-month follow-up period. There was a dramatic increase in citations issued for noncompliance of the state law in the experimental community and this ticketing behavior continued during the follow-up period. In contrast, virtually no tickets were issued in the control community over the entire 4.5-year period. Overall, police in the experimental community were 44 times more likely than those in the control community to enforce the safety seat law. The Lavelle et al. (1992) study illustrates how important it is to understand and resolve any administrative or personal barriers that may hinder enforcement of a new policy.

Drafting of Legislation

The way legislation is drafted can also be extremely important to the ultimate impact of any policy. Two examples can be offered to illustrate this point. On the positive side, in 1985, the Minnesota legislature increased the state tax on tobacco by 5 cents and used a portion of funds acquired by this new taxation to support school-based tobacco use prevention programs. Five years later, 96% of all school districts in Minnesota had applied for and received prevention program funding (Perry, Murray, & Griffin, 1990). In other words, the increased tobacco tax probably had some immediate effect on the consumption of tobacco products by young people, and then some of the new tax revenues was used to fund programs to further prevent tobacco use by school children.

On the negative side, Feighery et al. (1991) indicated that the way California legislation outlawing the sale of tobacco products to minors was written undermined its ultimate enforcement. Judges objected to two provisions of the California statute: (1) individuals would have a permanent criminal record because of a misdemeanor violation if found guilty in a court proceeding, and (2) the seller of the product, not the store manager or owner, had to pay the fine. As a result, merchants who refused to pay the required fine were treated leniently by judges in court. This example indicates the importance of carefully drafting the language of any new legislation and consulting first with the police and courts before the legislation is enacted to determine the feasibility of its enforcement.

INFLUENCING POLICY

The best way to create or influence social policy to achieve different ends is not known, but two strategies have met with success: top-down and bottom-up approaches.

Top-down Approaches

Top-down approaches involve consultation with those in authority such as legislators and agency or governmental administrators to initiate new policies or improve current ones. In other cases, attempts are made to influence policy at the highest level that in turn is expected to have a positive influence on policies and behavior at lower administrative levels. For example, the decision of the US Congress to link federal highway funds to a minimum legal drinking age of 21 is one example of a national policy that affected state policy, which in turn produced positive effects as described earlier.

Another example comes from Canada when in 1988 the Ministry of Education required that all local boards of education in the province of Ontario had to develop a comprehensive drug education and intervention policy and that the policy had to contain at least four major elements: a drug curriculum, an early intervention component to identify students with initial problems, counseling for those with more serious drug problems, and school disciplinary procedures relative to drug use (Gliksman, Allison, Adlaf, & Newton-Taylor, 1995). Many local schools already had policies in effect with regard to the latter two components, but not with respect to the first two, which emphasize prevention. Three years later, the Ministry of Education's provincial policy had a significant impact on local policies. The proportion of schools with an operational preventive curriculum more than doubled from 41 to 90%, and the number of early detection and intervention programs also doubled. The local schools' response to the Ministry of Education's new policy thus resulted in a substantial increase in primary and indicated prevention initiatives. The impact of these new prevention programs must be determined, of course, but their existence at a local level reflects a more comprehensive and systematic approach to drug use than had existed previously.

A good example of consultation with legislators to influence their policy decisions is the work of Fawcett, Seekins, and Jason (1987) who reported success in following a five-step process. These steps involved: (1) identifying those in a critical position to set policy; (2) understanding their interests; (3) determining the most relevant information; (4) collecting this information; and (5) reporting the information in a useful manner. The issue was an upcoming vote on a child passenger safety act that would require infants and young children to be placed in approved child safety devices when riding in motor vehicles. In a successful attempt to promote the passage of this legislation, Fawcett et al. (1987) proceeded through Coleman's (1972) five steps in two states: Kansas and Illinois.

In brief, Fawcett et al. learned that the relevant legislators needed credible data on two issues: (1) the social significance of the issue, and (2) the reaction of local citizens to the proposed legislation. Accordingly, both behavioral observational procedures to monitor the use of child safety seats and survey data were collected. The researchers presented data to legislators in both states regarding the low percentage of children who currently traveled in car safety seats and the high public support that existed for the proposed bill. In Kansas, there was the opportunity to present this information in public testimony before the state legislature and the presenters took care to be brief and clear and avoid scientific jargon. In Illinois, a controlled experiment was possible. Letters containing information on current car seat use and citizen's support for new legislation were sent to a randomly selected half of the state senators. These letters noted how many children in Illinois were killed or injured over the past few years and described the low percentage of current Illinois drivers correctly using child safety seats. The legislation was passed in both states. Whereas 79% of the Illinois state senators who received the researchers' letter subsequently voted for the legislation, only 53% of those who did not receive the letter did so. Fawcett et al. (1987) offered several useful suggestions for others wishing to become involved in influencing policy on social issues.

Bottom-up Approaches

Bottom-up approaches consist of efforts initiated by local citizens to develop more effective policies. Grass roots advocacy campaigns have been responsible for some major achievements. The Association for Retarded Citizens (ARC), a nationwide self-help group, played a major role in the passage of Public Law 94-142, the Education for All Handicapped Children Act, which has been expanded in several ways since its initial passage in 1975. Readers may not realize that PL 94-142 was passed to address a major educational injustice. Many schools throughout the country were failing to effectively educate children with various disabilities. Before passage of PL 94-142, the type of education given to children with special needs such as those with learning, developmental, or physical disabilities was at the total discretion of schools. Before passage of PL 94-142, it was estimated that 1 million students with various disabilities were excluded from public schools and at least 2 million more were not receiving the type of education they needed (Terman et al., 1996). National laws now guarantee the right to a free public education appropriate to one's needs and in the least restrictive environment possible for all children age 3–21. Many states also operate programs for children from birth to 3 years.

Mothers Against Drunk Drivers (MADD), a lay advocacy group, is generally credited for the passage of many drunk-driving laws throughout the United States and for changing social norms about drivers who drink (Bloch & Ungerleider, 1988). MADD effectively raised public consciousness and orchestrated an effective community campaign for tougher drunk-driving legislation, including increasing the minimum drinking age to 21. The positive consequences of such legislation have already been discussed. The success of groups such as ARC and MADD indicates that preventive action need not begin with professionals. Prevention is everybody's business.

Potential Problems

One potential problem with top-down approaches is the ineffective way local communities implement policies initiated at a higher level. For example, Chapter 1 (formerly Title I) created through the Education Consolidation and Improvement Act is the largest federal education program and serves approximately 5 million children. The federal government provides local school districts with money through Chapter 1 to educate children from low-income households. This policy makes good sense, since such children are at higher risk for educational problems (see Chapter 3, this volume). Unfortunately, Chapter 1 programs are not always implemented in ways that provide adequate assistance to low-income children. One field study (Rowan & Guthrie, 1989) found that children in Chapter 1 programs received only 10 extra minutes of help per day in reading and math. Other studies have found that low-income inner-city children spend 16% *less* time in active academic pursuits than children in suburban schools; first graders in one inner-city school averaged no more than 10 seconds a day of directed reading instruction (Carta, 1992). One cannot expect children at risk for academic problems to be successful following such superficial instruction.

As another example, boards of education in most states mandate their local school districts to conduct prevention programs in many areas such as AIDS and substance use, sexual abuse, and various health topics. Sometimes the content and duration of the program is specified (i.e., there must be 5 hours of instruction on sexual abuse) and at other times the schools have considerable freedom in meeting educational requirements. There are three major problems with this process. First, there is seldom any sound empirical basis for specific mandates (why 5 hours devoted to sexual abuse?). Second, schools seldom receive any help from state boards of education in choosing an appropriate and well-validated program. Third, there is usually no directive to evaluate any adopted program. As a result, many schools develop their own curricula without any outside consultation or choose commercially available programs that are the easiest to implement (brief informational programs) but which are unlikely to be successful in changing behavior. Many school prevention programs are thus put and kept in place not because they are effective, but because they satisfy bureaucratic requirements (Durlak, 1995).

Need for a Stronger Policy on Prevention

Prevention does not occupy a prominent place in the national policy of the United States. The allocation of resources is one useful way to gauge priorities. Only about 3% of all health care dollars in the United States are devoted to prevention (Levit, Lazenby, Letsch, & Cowan, 1991). These data clearly reflect how the current service philosophy places relatively little importance on prevention versus care for established problems. As a result, many prevention programs are not initiated with stable sources of administrative support and funding. History teaches us that lack of durable support will spell eventual doom for some prevention programs, regardless of their initial level of success (see Chapter 1, this volume). Future policies that develop secure administrative and financial support for prevention programming are vital in insuring the long-term viability of prevention.

SUMMARY

This chapter was an introduction to the importance of policy in shaping and influencing behavior. Current policy in the United States does not favor prevention. Only 3% of health care funding is devoted to prevention, while the remainder goes to treating established problems. Yet, there are several indications of how policy can be used in a total public health effort at prevention. For instance, since there is a negative relationship between the price and demand for products, taxes on tobacco and alcoholic products can be raised to decrease the use of these substances by young people. Passage of clean air (no-smoking) laws is also associated with diminished smoking among adolescents. Raising the legal age for drinking to age 21 has had the dual benefit of reducing drinking among teens and decreasing alcohol-related traffic fatalities.

Legislation should not be seen as a quick-fix solution to social problems. The content, implementation, and ecological fit of a policy are important. For example, most jurisdictions outlaw the sale of tobacco and alcoholic products to minors, yet many merchants regularly ignore such prohibitions unless the legislation is consistently enforced by local police and appropriate penalties are applied to merchants' behavior.

Two major strategies used in changing or modifying current policies are the top-down and bottom-up approaches. In the former, one hopes to influence policymakers to make decisions that will filter down to the target population. In the latter approach, local citizens initiate the movement to change policy. Mothers Against Drunk Driving and the Association for Retarded Citizens are two grass roots advocacy groups that have been responsible for some far-reaching positive social policy changes.

10

Current Status and Future Directions

INTRODUCTION

Previous chapters have summarized findings and discussed some issues germane to specific areas such as the prevention of behavioral and social problems, academic problems, and so on. The intent of this last chapter is to highlight some important findings and themes that have emerged across these different areas. In doing so, some liberties have been taken in synthesizing prevention research. Investigators have not used the same terminology or measurement procedures across studies, so some judgments and inferences have been made. Programs also vary greatly in their scope and focus, so there are exceptions to each of the following comments and recommendations. Although it is impossible to do justice to all of the prevention programs that have been discussed in earlier chapters, the following sections emphasize some important discoveries and principles that have emerged among diverse interventions. The first section summarizes the general outcomes of prevention, the second section offers some guidelines for improving interventions, and the final section offers a few comments on the future.

MAJOR RESEARCH FINDINGS

Prevention Works

It is clear that prevention works. There are many interventions that have enhanced the positive health and adjustment of children and adolescents, reduced the subsequent rate of problems, or achieved both

177

types of outcomes. With only one exception (the primary prevention of sexual abuse), positive results have been obtained in each area that has been reviewed: mental health, academics, physical health and sexuality, drug use, injuries, and physical abuse. Some of these areas contain many successful interventions and others contain fewer, but each has some exemplary programs, indicating that it is possible to help young people through preventive intervention. Moreover, both primary prevention, which attempts to preclude subsequent problems in currently normal populations, and indicated prevention (or secondary prevention), which is assistance for those with early signs of difficulties, have been effective.

Prevention Has Practical Benefits

In addition to the statistical significance that has been achieved in many research studies, there are many illustrations of the practical benefits of prevention. Several notable findings are summarized in Table 10.1 and illustrate quite dramatically how prevention has produced meaningful changes in the lives of children and adolescents.

For instance, studies in mental health have been able to reduce the future rate of clinical mood disorders in adolescents by 56% (Clarke et al., 1995), the proportion of children displaying clinical levels of aggression by 66% (Hawkins et al., 1991), and the proportion of children judged to have serious adjustment difficulties by 50% (Tremblay et al., 1992). Among drug studies, the future use of tobacco, marijuana, and alcohol have fallen by 38 to 45% (Hansen & Graham, 1991; Johnson et al. 1990; Perry et al., 1992). In the academic realm, preschool programs have reduced subsequent placements in special education classes by an average of 48%, reduced future grade retentions by 32%, and reduced school dropouts by 26% (Barnett, 1990). Some individual programs have reduced these negative outcomes by 67 to 90% (Campbell & Ramey, 1995; Knoff & Batsche, 1995).

In the general area of health, adolescent pregnancy rates have dropped by 30 to 41% (Allen et al., 1994; Zabin et al., 1986), adolescent sexual activity has been reduced by 37% (St. Lawrence et al., 1995), low-birth-weight infants have been reduced by 42% (Ershoff et al., 1990), and children have reduced their intake of sodium, saturated fats, and total fats by 47%, 25%, and 13%, respectively (Simons-Morton et al. 1988, 1991). Future rates of nonfatal injuries in children have fallen by 26 to 33% (Schelp, 1988; Schwartz et al., 1993). After their participation in some health promotion programs, children have begun exercising at levels recommended for good cardiovascular fitness (Kelder et al., 1993).

Table 10.1. Studies Illustrating Practical Benefits of Prevention

Area	Outcome[a]
Mental health	
Clarke et al. (1995)	56% fewer clinical mood disorders
Hawkins et al. (1991)	66% fewer children with clinical levels of aggression
Tremblay et al. (1992)	50% fewer children with serious adjustment difficulties and 50% more children well-adjusted
Olweus (1994)	50% less peer bullying
Drug use	
Perry et al. (1992)	39% fewer smokers
Johnson et al. (1990)	38% less marijuana use
Hansen & Graham (1991)	45% less alcohol use
Academics	
Barnett (1990)	14 preschool programs collectively reduced special education placements by 48%, future grade retentions by 32%, and school dropouts by 26%
Physical health and sexuality	
Ershoff et al. (1990)	42% fewer low-birth-weight infants
Girgis et al. (1993)	Children three times more likely to protect themselves against skin cancer
Kelder et al. (1993)	Children exercising at levels recommended for good cardiovascular fitness
Allen et al. (1994)	41% reduction in adolescent pregnancies
Simons-Morton et al. (1991)	Intake of sodium, saturated fats, and total fats reduced by 47%, 25%, and 13%, respectively
St. Lawrence et al. (1995)	37% reduction in adolescent sexual activity
Injuries and child maltreatment	
Olds et al. (1986)	50% reduction in child maltreatment
O'Malley & Wagenaar (1991)	26% reduction in alcohol-related traffic fatalities
Spiegel & Lindaman (1977)	35% reduction in deaths due to injuries[b]
Schelp (1988)	33% reduction in nonfatal injuries
Schwartz et al. (1993)	26% reduction in nonfatal injuries
Walton (1982)	75% reduction in fatal poisonings in young children[b]

[a]Most outcomes expressed in percentages were determined by comparing the relative status of experimental and control groups at postintervention or follow-up. If 20% of the experimental group and 40% of controls are aggressive, then the program has been successful in reducing the future rate of aggression by 50%.
[b]These data based on pre- and posttest changes occurring within the intervention group only.

and were three times more likely to practice behaviors that protect them again skin cancer (Girgis et al., 1993). Finally, in some cases, prevention has literally saved lives. Alcohol-related traffic fatalities have fallen by 26.3% (O'Malley & Wagenaar, 1991), deaths due to injuries by 35% (Spiegel & Lindaman, 1977), and fatal poisonings of young children by 75% (Walton, 1982).

Most of the studies in Table 10.1 are primary prevention programs involving normal populations, but indicated prevention (secondary prevention) has also yielded several noteworthy results. In several cases, target children's behavioral or academic functioning that was initially inferior to well-adjusted peers before intervention has become comparable to these same peers following intervention (Durlak & Gillespie, 1995; Forehand & Long, 1988; Greenwood et al., 1989). Such data imply that these target populations may no longer be at risk.

Not summarized in Table 10.1 are the findings indicating that prevention can be cost-effective. Prevention programs have returned $3.00 (Ginsberg & Silverberg, 1994), $8.00 (Barnett, 1993), $14.00 (Miller & Galbraith, 1995), or over $45.00 (Windsor et al., 1993) in benefits for every dollar spent. Furthermore, most current cost analyses have underestimated the full range of program effects, because many personal and social benefits from prevention such as reduced emotional pain and suffering and enhanced psychological well-being have not been considered (see Chapter 8).

In summary, prevention is clearly an idea whose time has come (Klein & Goldston, 1977). Prevention significantly improves the adjustment of young people and exerts a meaningful, practical impact on their lives. Among those studies collecting such information, program results have been durable over time and interventions have been cost-effective. The overall pattern of findings clearly indicates that more research and practice should be devoted to prevention. The currently distorted imbalance of spending only 3% of available money and resources on prevention while devoting the remainder to the treatment of established problems needs to change.

An Important Qualification

Prevention does not work all the time, forever, for everyone, and may not save money in every instance. Throughout this book I have highlighted programs that have been relatively well-designed and that have obtained good results. Every successful intervention has not been able to match the outcomes noted in Table 10.1. Nevertheless, model programs can inspire others by illustrating the potential of prevention and documenting what can be accomplished under the right conditions. An important challenge for future preventionists is clarifying under what circumstances prevention is most effective in order to determine the who, what, where, when, and why of prevention (Gullotta, 1994).

In the next section, findings in prevention are translated into some general guidelines for future programs. These suggestions may not apply in every case, but they are applicable across a wide range of interventions.

GUIDELINES FOR IMPROVING PROGRAMS

Implications from Risk Research

Current findings on risk factors suggest the importance of multilevel interventions in prevention and the need to adopt a comprehensive framework of health in program evaluations.

Need for Multilevel Interventions

Table 10.2 lists the prominent risk factors targeted in interventions designed to prevent eight major negative outcomes. Not every risk factor for each outcome has been included, some factors are highly related (e.g., low socioeconomic and impoverished neighborhoods), and it is not possible to prioritize the relative importance of different risk factors for different outcomes. Nevertheless, Table 10.2 suggests that multilevel interventions are needed in prevention. There is no negative outcome in Table 10.2 that is related to risk at only one level of analysis and some outcomes are associated with risks present at all five levels (e.g., drug use and school failure). Indeed, many of the programs discussed in previous chapters have intervened at multiple levels (individual and family, school and peer, and so on), and a few programs have intervened at all five levels. In other words, exemplary programs in prevention seem able to intervene at multiple levels of influence to target the multiple risk factors that exist at these levels. Approaches restricted to a single level of intervention may have much more limited impact, presumably because they cannot modify as many risk factors relevant to the targeted outcome.

Need for a Comprehensive Approach to Health

The need for a comprehensive approach becomes apparent as one examines the interrelationship among the risk factors in Table 10.2.

Table 10.2. Risk Factors for Eight Major Outcomes

Level of analysis	Outcome							
	Behavior problems	School failure	Poor physical health	Physical injury	Physical abuse	Pregnancy	Drug use	AIDS
Community								
1. Impoverished neighborhood[a]	X	X	X	X	X	X	X	
2. Ineffective social policy[b]	X	X	X		X	X	X	
School								
1. Poor school quality[c]	X	X	X			X	X	X
Peer								
1. Peer pressure/influence regarding negative or high-risk behavior	X	X	X	X		X	X	X
Family								
1. Low socioeconomic status	X	X	X	X	X	X	X	X
2. Parental problems (depression, anxiety, drug abuse)	X	X	X	X	X	X	X	X
3. Child-rearing practices	X	X	X	X	X		X	

Individual level

1. Early onset of target problem	X	X	X	X	X	X[f]
2. Problems in another area	X	X	X	X	X	X

Other

1. Stress[e]	X	X	X	X	X	X

[a] A combination of negative social indicators such as lack of available jobs, high rates of crime and violence, inadequate social services, a transient population, few social ties among residents, and negative views about the community.

[b] That is, policies that limit access to needed services, or are inconsistently applied or poorly implemented, or that allow access to products such as tobacco or alcohol.

[c] Can be reflected by low academic expectations, poor leadership, insufficient attention to basic skills, and poor teacher–principal–parent relationships.

[d] Most often, inconsistency, punitiveness, lack of warmth or nurturance, and modeling of negative behaviors such as poor health care practices.

[e] Stress can occur at any level of analysis and affect youth directly or indirectly through its impact on adults and peers.

[f] Early sexual activity is a risk factor.

Note. All relevant risk factors for each outcome are not presented.

Several risk factors apply to many possible outcomes. For example, the following factors are related to six or more of the eight negative outcomes noted in Table 10.2: living in an impoverished neighborhood, ineffective social policies, poor school quality, negative peer modeling, parental child-rearing practices, low socioeconomic status, early onset of the target problem, and problems in other areas. Therefore, it comes as no surprise that interventions with different goals have nevertheless targeted an overlapping set of risk factors.

At the same time, it is also noteworthy that the appearance of one negative outcome is often a risk factor for the appearance of additional difficulties in other areas. Table 10.3 presents further general information on the relationship among negative outcomes and illustrates the notion that most problems appear not in isolation but in conjunction with other problems. In other words, most maladapting children and adolescents have multiple rather than singular adjustment problems; if one problem appears, then young people are usually at risk for other problems as well, at least among the outcomes listed in Table 10.3. The causal connections among multiple problems are not known, and it is not possible to explicate all the possible interrelationships among negative outcomes. Two examples can be provided. (1) The appearance of academic difficulties is often associated with externalizing and internalizing problems, poor peer relations, drug use, and adolescent pregnancy. (2) The use of alcohol places youth at risk for death or serious injury from automobile crashes and increases the likelihood of early sexual activity and unprotected sexual intercourse.

The data from Tables 10.2 and 10.3 thus support the following logical argument: If different negative outcomes share several risk factors, and if one negative outcome that is prevented is a risk factor for other outcomes, then preventive programs should be able to simultaneously prevent multiple negative outcomes. This should occur according to the relative weight or influence of the risk factors that are modified in the intervention.[1]

For instance, if poor school quality is a risk factor for academic difficulties and also plays a role in drug use, adolescent pregnancy rates, and some mental health problems, then improving school quality should not only directly affect academic achievement but also impact these other adjustment domains. Similarly, poor physical health puts children at risk for a variety of academic, mental health, and social

[1]The same reasoning can be extended to prevention as health promotion, although we have less empirical information on the relationships among competencies across different outcome domains.

Table 10.3. Elaboration of How One Negative Outcome Is a Risk Factor for Other Outcomes

If this problem is present:	Populations are also at increased risk for							
	Behavior problems[a]	School failure	Physical health problems	Physical injury	Physical abuse	Pregnancy	Drug use	AIDS
Behavior problem		X		X	X	X	X	X
School failure	X			X	X	X	X	X
Physical health problems	X	X		X	X	X	X	X
Physical injury	X	X	X		X		X	
Physical abuse	X	X	X	X			X	
Adolescent pregnancy	X	X	X				X	
Drug use	X	X	X			X		X

[a]Either externalizing (e.g., aggression) or internalizing problems (e.g., depression, anxiety).

problems; improving physical health should have some impact on these other areas.

Can multiple problems be prevented with a single intervention? The answer is "Yes." Some of the most exciting findings in prevention have come from programs that have produced positive effects in different domains of functioning. For instance, some successful academic programs have also significantly reduced behavioral problems or drug use, or improved social functioning and peer relations (Barnett, 1990; Knoff & Batsche, 1995; Stevens & Slavin, 1995); some physical health programs have had similar effects (Infant and Health Development Program, 1990; Olds & Kitzman, 1993); and some mental health programs have produced significant positive changes in academic performance and peer relations (Durlak & Wells, 1997a,b). Such data indicate that intervention can prevent multiple problems.

Unfortunately, most investigators have been remiss in examining such possibilities and have restricted their evaluations to only one domain of functioning: academics, or physical health, or mental health. In effect, across the more than 1200 outcome studies conducted to date, preventionists have probably underestimated the true positive effects of prevention by failing to consider and evaluate whether or not programs successful in one area also have some positive impact in other areas of functioning.

Nevertheless, the success of some programs indicates that it is important to have a comprehensive view of health in mind when planning program evaluations in order to assess all the possible outcomes that might reasonably occur. Figure 10.1 presents one potentially useful model of health. The model accommodates both a health promotion and a problem-focused orientation. First, the broad construct of healthy functioning is broken down into four main components: psychological, physical, social, and academic health. Second, each of these four components is further subdivided in terms of both possible problems and competencies (the latter being consistent with a health promotion focus). As mentioned in Chapter 1, positive health is not simply the absence of problems, but rather the presence of adaptive or positive skills or characteristics. Finally, each of the eight areas of health has a number of subcomponents, only some of which have been identified in Fig. 10.1. For instance, in the area of mental health, one can assess the presence of problems (e.g., levels of aggression or depression) as well as the presence of positive skills or competencies (e.g., decision making, self-control); there is also a competency and problem side to each of the other areas of health.

Each individual variable listed in Fig. 10.1 is a legitimate primary target for prevention and additional goals can be added. What is essential to realize, however, is the interconnectedness among the dimen-

A MODEL OF HEALTH

PHYSICAL DOMAIN

HEALTH	PROBLEMS
Physical Indices: muscle tone, cholesterol level, blood pressure body weight. Behaviors: eating patterns nutritional intake, exercise levels	Various medical problems and illnesses Developmental disabilities Physical injury Sexually transmitted diseases HIV/AIDS Adolescent Pregnancy

PSYCHOLOGICAL DOMAIN

HEALTH	PROBLEMS
Well-being Self-efficacy High Self-esteem Adaptive skills: coping, self-control goal-setting, decision-making	Clinical disorders Subclinical-level problems Drug Misuse Violence, delinquency Risky behaviors: driving after drinking, not using seat belts, unprotected intercourse

SOCIAL DOMAIN

HEALTH	PROBLEMS
Peer acceptance Altruism Friendships and bonds with others Effective social skills: communication, problem-solving conflict-resolution, assertiveness	Peer rejection Social isolation Social anxiety

ACADEMIC DOMAIN

HEALTH	PROBLEMS
Full development of cognitive abilities Ability to work with others Metalearning (learning how to learn)	Academic deficiencies Grade retention Placement in special education Test anxiety School Dropouts

Figure 10.1. Possible targets for prevention in the four domains of health.

sions of health. Physical, mental, social, and academic health are frequently related. Evaluators should consider how to assess possible outcomes in the four major domains noted in Fig. 10.1, in recognition of the relationships that exist among these domains.

For example, the placement of some items is rather arbitrary. Adolescent pregnancy is listed as a physical health problem because of the medical risk to mother and infant, but adolescent mothers and their offspring are at risk for a variety of social, educational, physical, and mental health problems (Furstenberg et al., 1987). Physical abuse is listed under the physical problems category, but also has possible negative ramifications for academic, social, and mental health. The implication is that interventions that reduce the incidence of adolescent pregnancy or physical child abuse are likely to affect other aspects of health as well. These possible effects need to be captured in program evaluations to gain a more complete assessment of the impact of prevention.

Emphasize Protective and Positive Factors

Another major implication from prevention research is that future interventions should concentrate on those factors that may be particularly important in protecting against negative outcomes (protective factors) or enhancing positive health (positive factors). Table 10.4 lists several variables that merit consideration because of their presence in many successful interventions. More research is needed to identify precisely what mechanisms operate to reduce negative outcomes (protective factors) or enhanced health (positive factors), and other variables may be added to the list in Table 10.4.

Each of the factors in Table 10.4 is discussed separately, although it must be kept in mind that protective–positive factors can interact with each other and with risk factors, and that each factor may be more or less important, depending on the specific outcome. This is simply another way of saying there is no single factor that by itself guards against all possible negative outcomes or is responsible for decidedly positive outcomes (i.e., enhanced health). Moving from the individual to the community level of analysis and intervention, the following factors are noteworthy.

Various Personal Skills

The acquisition of a variety of coping and adaptive skills is often associated with positive program outcomes. The skills most commonly targeted relate to communication and self-control, goal setting and deci-

Table 10.4. Variables Meriting Further Consideration as Protective or Positive Factors

Level of analysis	Factor
1. Individual	Various personal and social skills

The most frequently targeted skills have related to communication, self-control, problem solving, goal setting and decision making, assertiveness, active coping, and self-monitoring skills.

2. Family	A good parent–child relationship

Elements of a good parent–child relationship include a positive bond between parent and child, parental understanding and sensitivity, careful monitoring and supervision of child behavior, and consistently applied child-rearing techniques that are more supportive and reinforcing than punitive.

3. Peer group	Peer modeling and support

Peer influence is particularly important with respect to drug taking, sexual activity, delinquency, and school performance.

4. School	Good academic performance

Multiple factors operate to enhance academic performance such as intensive preschool programs that prepare at-risk children for school entry, well-organized and administered school programs that encourage students to attain high levels of performance, and strong collaborative relationships among principals, teachers, students, and parents.

5. Community	Social support

Social support can buffer against stress, reinforce and thus maintain newly acquired adaptive skills, and contribute directly to psychological well-being.

Norms promoting prevention

If norms promoting prevention are obvious in a setting, if important community members model normative behavior, and if reinforcements and sanctions are consistently delivered to behaviors that conform to or violate the norms, respectively, then more preventive behaviors will occur among individuals in that setting.

Note. A protective factor reduces the likelihood of a negative outcome while a positive factor increases the likelihood of a decidedly positive outcome such as enhanced psychological well-being.

sion making, assertiveness, and various coping and self-monitoring skills. Furthermore, it is clear that systematic skills training, is necessary to help young people acquire these skills. Merely telling young people how to behave differently will not have much effect. A social learning paradigm is often used in skills training, and Appendix A provides an overview of the steps involved in effective training programs. Allensworth (1993) has summarized the literature on skills training very well by noting: "Acquisition of basic skills at appropriate ages appears to be a primary component of all prevention" (p. 17).

Parent–Child Relationship

Many programs strive to improve the parent–child relationship, which can be accomplished in different ways depending on the family situation. For instance, during infancy attention may be directed at fostering a secure attachment bond between parent and child (e.g., van de Boom, 1995). As the child grows, parents can be taught developmentally appropriate child care and child-rearing practices. The ultimate goals of many family interventions are often twofold: (1) to help parents become more sensitive to and understanding of their children's developmental needs, and (2) to guide parents to act more positively and less punitively toward their children. In addition, some programs specifically seek to empower parents to be more effective self-advocates and help seekers.

Peer Modeling and Reinforcement

Peer modeling and reinforcement has been another feature of many successful programs. Positive peer behavior and pressure can be particularly important in influencing behavior related to drug taking, sexual activity, delinquency, and academic performance. Using credible, high-status peers in an intervention is a way of modeling preventive behavior and giving support or reinforcement to those who imitate such behaviors. Using peers as change agents has the double benefit of taking advantage of the helper therapy principle (Riessman, 1965) which emphasizes that people often benefit from helping others. As noted in Chapter 3, for example, tutoring is an effective form of academic instruction, and in some cases tutors have benefited more than their tutees.

Good Academic Performance

There is also growing evidence that good school performance can protect children against various negative social and behavioral outcomes, such as psychological problems related to depression, low self-esteem and externalizing behaviors, peer difficulties, adolescent pregnancy, and drug use. As noted in Chapter 3, several investigators have independently added academic components to interventions designed to prevent social and behavioral problems in recognition of the importance of academic achievement in children's lives. The academic health of target populations should not be overlooked.

Social Norms Promoting Prevention

It also appears that the existence of social norms favoring prevention can be a protective–positive factor. In general, norms favoring prevention are not prominent in American society. Some cross-cultural comparisons illustrate this point in terms of the extent to which different cultures respond to preventive interventions. For example, with respect to the wearing of protective headgear such as bicycle helmets, interventions conducted in the United States are considered successful when they can increase rates of compliance from 10% to around 30% (see Chapter 6). In contrast, compliance with helmet laws in countries such as Israel and Spain often exceeds 85% (Ballart & Riba, 1995; Ginsberg & Silverberg, 1994).

Norms typically do not produce quick changes, but tend to exercise their effect slowly and cumulatively over time. Some individuals are initially affected; their behavioral change then influences others and the pool of individuals affected by new norms slowly increases over time, creating a widening ripple effect throughout the population. This means that long-term evaluations may be needed to allow sufficient time for norms to change and to influence behavior (see below). For example, positive normative changes regarding drug taking appeared after 3 years in Project Northland (Perry et al., 1996).

Norms can have a strong effect on behavior if they are well articulated and obvious in a setting, if important members of the community (e.g., teachers, parents, and peers) model behaviors consistent with the norms, and if individuals receive encouragement and reinforcement for behavior that conforms to the norms.

Social Support

Social support is another construct that deserves consideration as a protective factor. Research suggests that social support can buffer individuals against the negative effects of stress and can be strongly related to positive aspects of well-being (Meehan, Durlak, & Bryant, 1993; Vaux, 1988). Social support has been a part of many family-oriented programs, has been provided by teachers and peers in school-based interventions, and has also been a feature of several transition interventions for children undergoing divorce, school change and entry, and stressful medical and dental procedures. The impact of social support is likely to vary as a function of what type of support is offered, by whom and when, and how satisfied recipients are with the support that is available (Vaux,

1988). These dimensions need to be carefully assessed in future interventions in an attempt to pinpoint the contribution of social support to program outcomes.

There are several other recommendations that can be offered to guide future prevention efforts. Once again, these comments do not apply in every circumstance, but they do have wide applicability.

Begin from a Sound Theoretical and Empirical Base

Most successful programs have a specific theory or a set of conceptions that guides the intervention. Theory helps in selecting a target population, composing the elements of the intervention, and deciding how to evaluate the program and interpret its results. Effective interventions are also driven by past empirical findings indicating that an approach is potentially effective and suggesting ways to test specific hypotheses.

Involve Parents as Much as Possible

Parents can play a critical role as positive role models and supportive and reinforcing figures in the lives of their children. Therefore, it is not surprising that many successful programs to prevent social and behavioral problems, drug use, and to improve academic functioning and physical health have involved parents. Parental involvement appears to be as important for older children and adolescents as it is in interventions for infants and preschoolers.

There have been difficulties encountered in securing the full participation of parents in prevention programs particularly if the program requires attendance at meetings offered at school or in the evenings. Offering home- or work-based interventions may be one good way to involve more parents (see below). Nevertheless, Schinke (1994) is correct in noting that "... little is known about ways to galvanize family members into preventive action in a predictably effective manner" (p. 50).

Abandon the Use of Information-Only Programs

We know what does not work in prevention. Programs that rely on informational strategies to change behavior have not been effective in any area of prevention in which they have been tried. In fact, the evidence is overwhelming that such programs do not significantly change behavior.

The use of information-only programs in prevention should be abandoned. These types of programs are still used because they are brief, easy to administer, and thus relatively inexpensive to operate, and their existence may satisfy administrative or social pressures to do something about prevention. However, informational programs provide a false sense of security that prevention is being accomplished when it is not. With a brief, didactically oriented program, schools, community, and governmental agencies can claim that they are doing prevention when, in reality, they are wasting valuable time and resources that could be better spent doing something more effective. This statement may seem harsh, but it is well-supported by current outcome research.

Compare Alternative Programs

In the early stages of a science it is customary to compare an experimental intervention to a no-treatment control group to answer the general question: Is the intervention better than nothing at all? The results of over 1200 outcome studies have answered this question affirmatively. Participants in a prevention program are generally better off than those who receive no program at all. Outcome data also suggest that prevention produces few negative side effects (Durlak & Wells, 1997a,b).

Comparisons of alternative programs are now needed. These comparisons should be addressed at providing information on what type of program produces what results for which members of the target population at what cost? Progress in prevention will be greatly fostered as we discover the relative advantages and limitations of different types of interventions.

Adopt a Long-Term Perspective

It takes time to view the full effects of prevention. Results from the Perry Preschool Program (Schweinhart & Weikart, 1988) indicated that intervention conducted when children were 3 to 4 years old subsequently reduced rates of adolescent delinquency 14 to 15 years later. This striking finding would not have been discovered without the patient long-term follow-up work of researchers. All program evaluations cannot be expected to follow samples for such a long period, but some follow-up is needed to assess how program participants fare over time.

Be Flexible in Providing Services

Programs are often conducted with the assumption that all participants should receive all parts of a program in a prescribed order and for the same period of time (e.g., everyone will participate once a week for 1 hour for 12 weeks and receive all three components of the program). This procedure is efficient if all participants truly need each program component and if all can benefit equally from the same amount of program exposure. In contrast, several successful interventions have individualized services according to need. This program flexibility has occurred most prominently in home-based services directed at physical health promotion and child maltreatment, academic programs, and in some injury prevention efforts. Individualized interventions have strong ecological validity, that is, that are well-matched to each family or child situation and are a wise use of available resources. Those that need more help and more services can receive them while those with fewer or different needs can also be accommodated.

Some programs (e.g., Forehand & Long, 1988) consist of a graded sequence of activities, but allow participants to proceed at their own pace. Some spend more time on some sections than others and complete the program at different rates. This is another way to match the program to participants' needs.

Pay Careful Attention to Program Implementation

Implementation generally refers to how well a proposed program is actually put into practice. There can be quite a gap between the type of program that is conceived and what actually occurs when the program is conducted in real-life settings. For instance, in school-based interventions, teachers may independently make their own judgments about what part or parts of the program to administer; they may omit portions of the program they do not agree with or that are more difficult to administer, or abandon the program completely if no one is available to help with any implementation problems that may occur.

Studies have consistently demonstrated the importance of program implementation. Either programs do not produce any significant positive effects unless they are well-implemented, or the amount of change achieved is directly related to the quality of program implementation (Durlak, 1995; Durlak & Ferrari, 1997).

Five strategies are often helpful in enhancing program implementation: (1) insuring that program practices and goals are acceptable to the host community; (2) carefully training those who will deliver the program so that they are able to conduct the program as planned; (3) "manualizing" the program so that its key elements can be replicated by other adopting agencies; (4) having mechanisms in place for ongoing monitoring of program implementation; and (5) remaining available for continual consultation and problem solving.

Expand Possible Sites for Prevention

The majority of prevention programs, approximately 75%, have been school based. School programs should continue, but more prevention should occur in other environments such as health care settings, community agencies, day care centers, the home, and the workplace.

For instance, there are more than 17,000 community-based organizations that already offer some services to youth such as chapters of Big Brothers/Big Sisters of America, YWCA and YMCA, and local churches, parks, and recreational departments (Carnegie Corporation, 1992). A few of these, such as the Junior League and Boys and Girls Clubs of America, have either sponsored some of the effective prevention programs discussed in earlier chapters (Philliber & Allen, 1992; St. Pierre et al., 1992), or have been a part of communitywide initiatives. For the most part, however, the potential and resources of community-based organizations in offering prevention programs are largely untapped. Community-based organizations can be an excellent home for prevention because of the support they receive from business and civic leaders and the vast volunteer pool available to many groups. Community-based organizations thus offer potential stability and administrative support for prevention and their collective lobbying efforts can influence policy and funding priorities.

The large growth in single-parent families and the need for both spouses to work in two-parent homes mean that creative strategies must be used to link services to target populations. An 8-to-5 office schedule of delivering services will miss too many people and evening programs may not appeal to families with limited time and resources. One approach to service delivery that has been very effective is home-based care. This has worked with respect to reducing academic and physical health problem, childhood injury and maltreatment, and some social and behavioral problems (see Chapters 2, 3, 5–7). Integrating prevention into routine health care appointments is another promising approach (see Chapters 5 and 6). Another possibility is to bring services into the workplace so that parents can participate. Corporations are willing to sponsor family-oriented worksite programs and their employees attend such programs (e.g., Colan et al., 1994; Felner et al., 1994).

Use a Collaborative Approach

Collaboration can take many different forms, but often it refers to a working relationship that combines inputs from three distinct groups: (1) those wishing to introduce an intervention into a setting, (2) those in community organizations and agencies who will host and perhaps

conduct the program, and (3) the potential consumers or program participants. A variety of strategies have been used to reach mutually satisfac-
tory agreements among these groups about what type of services will be
provided and how they will offered.

There are several potential benefits to a collaborative approach.
Collaboration (1) provides outsiders with a better understanding of local
needs and priorities, (2) can uncover and capitalize on community
strengths and resources, (3) may be particularly important in developing
culturally appropriate interventions for different populations, (4) increases the community's sense of ownership of the program, which
increases the likelihood the program will be maintained over time, and
(5) helps to create and emphasize social norms promoting prevention.

Work with Community Coalitions

The growing recognition that multiple environmental and social
forces influence behavior underscores the need to mount communitywide initiatives. "History teaches us that organized community
effort to prevent disease and promote health is both valuable and effective" (Institute of Medicine, 1988, p. 17). Working with community
coalitions further emphasizes the necessity for collaboration and coordination among multiple disciplines.

One format for community coalitions is the Healthy Cities Model,
which has become a worldwide movement directed at social change to
promote health and prevent disease. Healthy Cities began in 1986 as a
World Health Organization plan targeting five to eight European cities.
The idea caught on rapidly and 4 years later included three international networks encompassing hundreds of cities (Flynn & Rains, 1993).

The basic idea of Healthy Cities is to place health high on the
city's agenda, to develop and implement specific plans to improve the
city's health using a coalition of governmental and local leaders, and to
find the resources to make the plans happen. Healthy Cities projects
typically involve a number of tasks: (1) reducing inequalities in health
status; (2) developing sound public health policies at the local level;
(3) creating physical and social environments that support health;
(4) strengthening community action for health; (5) helping people develop new health-related skills; and (6) reorienting health services to be
supportive of the principles of health promotion.

Community coalitions vary along several dimensions including
their primary goals. In addition to Healthy Cities, which focuses primarily on physical health issues, there are now over 2000 community
coalitions targeting the use of alcohol, tobacco, and other drugs (Falco,

1992). Coalitions can become very complex organizations. Project Freedom, which has had some success in preventing substance abuse, involved over 750 individuals from almost 100 different organizations (Fawcett et al., 1996). As a result of their complexity and diversity, researchers are just beginning to understand some of the processes and outcomes of coalitions (Fetterman, Kafterian, & Wandersman, 1995).

Preliminary data indicate that successful community-based projects are effective in accomplishing several critical tasks. These tasks include formulating clear and realistic goals, reaching consensus on priorities, developing specific action plans to reach goals, and securing the resources needed (e.g., computer assistance or technical knowledge) to accomplish different tasks (DeAngelis, 1996). These findings suggest ways that preventionists can provide assistance to community-based coalitions.

Use Mass Media and Technology Effectively

Early public health efforts to use the mass media did not usually meet with much success because these campaigns were founded on faulty assumptions and were poorly implemented. Many early media campaigns emphasized public service announcements (PSAs) that were used to pass on information about current scientific findings and to recommend new health practices. Such an approach is unlikely to lead to much behavior change. Moreover, the distribution of PSAs often depended on the good will of the media industry who were not energetic in promoting public health. Public health groups depended on free time from television and PSAs were often run at times when audience reach and impact were low (i.e., in the early morning hours). In addition, PSAs were not very sophisticated or polished, and thus suffered in appeal and interest compared to paid television programming and advertising.

Mass media campaigns have changed dramatically in theory and execution over the past few years, with a corresponding increase in their effectiveness. Now most experts believe that mass media efforts can be successful in changing behavior, particularly when they are theory driven, sustained and intensive, use sound social marketing strategies, adopt realistic goals, and are complemented by community action strategies and interpersonal approaches. The latter might include policy initiatives, creating new skill-building and social support health programs, or making low-cost self-help materials available (Backer, Rogers & Sopory, 1992; Flay, 1987).

Media advocacy is an emerging technique with much preventive merit. Media advocacy is a combination of science, politics, and activism:

> The purpose of media advocacy is to use the media strategically to apply pressures for changes in policy to promote public health goals. It provides a framework for moving the public health discussion from a primary focus on the health behaviors of the individual to behaviors of policymakers and corporate executives whose decisions structure the environment in which individual health decisions are made.... Media advocacy is a tactic for community group to communicate their own story in their own words to promote social change. (Wallack, Dorfman, Jernigan & Themba, 1993, p. xi).

Mothers Against Drunk Driving is probably the group best known for its effective media advocacy efforts, but Wallack et al. (1993) describe several other success stories.

Finally, preventionists should consider how technology can advance prevention. For example, the increasing sophistication of interactive computer systems holds promise for reaching large segments of the population. As another example, Winett and colleagues have reported success in using home videos to improve family communication and discussion about HIV/AIDS (Winett & Anderson, 1994).

Combine Qualitative and Quantitative Strategies

Although this book has emphasized quantitative findings, the qualitative aspects of prevention should not be overlooked. Several different types of qualitative approaches have been used by preventionists such as interviews, focus groups, team meetings, community forums, and problem-solving and brainstorming sessions. Qualitative methods can be extremely helpful in gauging the appropriateness of a proposed program and in making necessary adjustments if needed, resolving problems related to program implementation and lack of community support, and understanding participants' reactions in order to improve the intervention or make it more appealing to more of the target population.

Offer More Comprehensive Interventions

Most prevention programs are categorical in nature, focusing on one major problem or outcome, such as drugs or academics. As the previous discussion suggests, however, there is much overlap in some of the basic features of prevention (what risk and protective factors are emphasized) and much potential overlap in program outcomes given that different components of health are often related. Therefore, there is a need to combine multidisciplinary resources and expertise and offer interventions that intentionally seek to achieve multiple goals. Such interventions would add conceptual and developmental continuity to the myriad of preventive offerings that now exist. For example, several preventive school programs are now offered in different grades to achieve different goals (e.g., to prevent drug use or to improve social skills) without much coordination or integration and all these programs exist independently from any concurrent medical efforts to improve health, community-based programs to reduce injury, or policy initiatives designed to achieve different ends.

A comprehensive approach means that professionals must transcend traditional turf issues to develop solid working relationships with colleagues in other disciplines. In other words, just as collaboration between professionals and community members are important, so is collaboration among the many professional disciplines involved in prevention. Professionals must come to realize that joining forces rather than proceeding independently is more likely to improve the economy and impact of prevention and to produce interventions that speak more effectively to the multiple needs of young people and their families. Funding agencies also need to be convinced of the value of comprehensive over categorical approaches and need to be willing to let preventionists devote their resources to achieving multiple ends.

THE FUTURE OF PREVENTION

In large part, the future of prevention depends on how well current systemic and personal barriers to prevention can be overcome. The major systemic barrier is the problem-oriented focus of the United States health care system, which devotes 98% of its resources to treating problems and only 3% to prevention (Levit et al., 1991). As a result, prevention programs are often insufficiently staffed and funded, providers in the general health care system are not reimbursed for preventive services, and prevention does not become a prominent service value. It is not easy to change such a system, so that attempts at many levels are needed. Increased funding for prevention is certainly one way to insure that more prevention is attempted.

Others have emphasized the need for more education and training (Moser, McCance & Smith, 1991; Price, 1986). Although continuing education workshops and specialized training programs have their place, over the long term perhaps the best way to increase the amount of prevention that occurs is to insure that all new professionals are well trained in prevention. During their professional careers, people tend to do what they are comfortable doing and have some experience with, which is often a reflection of how they were initially trained. The training period is also a critical time when primary values and priorities develop. What is important to my field and what type of (doctor, psychologist, educator) do I want to be?

Therefore, the multiple disciplines related to prevention should require training in prevention for all their students. Such training should involve both theory and practice that is provided through coursework, practica, and mentoring experiences. The natural objection to this suggestion is that there is no room in current professional curricula to add prevention training: "What would we take out? We have no room." This is, of course, a deceptive response. There is always room for essential things.

For instance, the American Academy of Pediatrics has recommended that the prevention of childhood injuries become integrated into all primary health care settings, suggesting that prevention is one standard of competence in its field (see Bass et al., 1993). Such a position implies that pediatric training programs should accommodate to this new training standard. Corresponding prevention-oriented requirements can be developed for other disciplines. As another example, surveys of the membership and leadership of the American Psychological Association indicate that prevention is one priority in the field's future (Oakland, 1994). Professional psychology programs, which usually do not provide much training in prevention, will have to be quickly restructured to insure that their new graduates acquire prevention-related skills.

If all new professionals received a thorough grounding in prevention, then they probably would do more prevention during their professional careers. They would also have more knowledge about which types of programs are likely to work, be in a more informed position to evaluate proposed interventions, and be more likely to advocate for prevention.

Concluding Comments

There is a danger in overselling prevention. The field will inevitably encounter some setbacks whenever program evaluations produce nonsignificant findings. Prevention will not be able to eliminate all future problems or be successful in every situation or for everyone. Therefore, it is important to view findings from individual studies in context. Negative results should challenge us to search for the factors that maximize program impact and efficiency. Current outcome data justify the position that prevention should be a prominent part in the array of services available to children and families. In some cases, well-timed and executed preventive programs may be all the assistance that some segments of the population will need. If we are truly interested in the development of our young people, we cannot afford to ignore the potential of prevention.

SUMMARY

Well-done outcome studies indicate that prevention works. Many interventions have significantly enhanced the positive health and adjustment of children and adolescents, reduced the subsequent rates of problems, or achieved both types of outcomes. Positive results have been obtained for different aspects of mental and physical health, drug use, academic performance, childhood injuries, and physical abuse and neglect. A few outstanding programs have reduced future problems by 30 to 50% or more. Problems in multiple domains can be positively affected by the same intervention, and an overlapping group of risk and protective factors is frequently targeted in interventions.

These developments suggest that a conceptual framework acknowledging the connections among physical, mental, social, and academic health should be adopted when designing and evaluating prevention programs and that more multidisciplinary collaboration and coordination are needed to offer more comprehensive programs. Several other suggestions for improving future interventions were offered. It is particularly important that professional training programs be restructured so that all students acquire prevention-related values, knowledge, and skills.

Appendix A

Characteristics of Effective Skill Training Programs

Many successful training programs use a social learning paradigm to teach new skills and behaviors. These programs often have the following elements:

1. Identify what skills or combination of skills will be taught.
2. Define each skill in clear operational terms so that progress on each skill can be carefully assessed.
3. Use a step-by-step training approach by focusing on one skill at a time and by breaking down complicated skills into more manageable components.
4. Clearly explain what the skill is and why it is important.
5. Demonstrate the effective use of each skill by using live and/or filmed models. Adult or peer models or both may be used.
6. Ask trainees to practice the modeled skill.
7. Give immediate performance feedback emphasizing positive reinforcement as much as possible.
8. Allow discussion of problems in skill acquisition so advice and guidance can be individualized to help each trainee.
9. Emphasize peer support during training; trainees can help each other learn the skills, so that group training is preferred over individual training.
10. Repeat steps 4 through 9 until sufficient skill mastery is achieved. Some training programs give homework assignments to increase the use and application of skills in the natural environment.
11. Move on to another skill by beginning again at step 4.
12. Improve the likelihood of skill maintenance by developing

sources of continuing support and reinforcement of newly learned skills. This can be done by involving peers, teachers, and parents in the intervention and by enacting new school and community policies.

13. Booster training sessions conducted at various follow-up periods are sometimes used to maintain skill mastery.

The above training approach is adaptable and efficient. Depending on the number and complexity of the skill(s), training takes from 4 to 20 hours and can develop proficiency in the following areas: communication and assertiveness, friendship making, safe sex, interpersonal problem solving and decision making, goal setting, relaxation and other stress reduction procedures, and different types of self-management practices related to self-instruction, self-monitoring, and self-reinforcement.

The same procedures can be used to train trainers; that is, to teach parents, teachers, older peers, college students, and others how to help children and adolescents acquire prevention-related skills. Several good sources discuss training strategies and provide examples (Cartledge & Milburn, 1980; Elliott & Gresham, 1993; Ladd & Mize, 1983; Stephens, 1978).

Appendix B

Helpful Resources on Prevention

BOOKS

The following texts on prevention are all highly recommended. These references typically describe numerous interventions and address many theoretical, research, and practical issues related to prevention.

Bloom, M. (1996). *Primary prevention practices.* Thousand Oaks, CA: Sage.

Cowen, E. L., Hightower, A. D., Pedro-Carroll, J. L., Work, W. C., & Wyman, P. A. (1996). *School-based prevention for children at risk: The Primary Mental Health Project.* Washington, DC: American Psychological Association.

Dryfoos, J. G. (1990). *Adolescents at risk: Prevalence and prevention.* New York: Oxford University Press.

Durlak, J. A. (1995). *School-based prevention programs for children and adolescents.* Thousand Oaks, CA: Sage.

Felner, R. D., Jason, L. A., Moritsugu, J. N., & Farber, S. S. (1983). *Preventive psychology: Theory, research and practice.* New York: Pergamon.

Glenwick, D. S., & Jason, L. A. (Eds.). (1993). *Promoting health and mental health in children, youth, and families.* New York: Springer.

Kessler, M., Goldston, S. E., & Joffe, J. M. (Eds.). (1992). *The present and future of prevention.* Newbury Park, CA: Sage.

Institute of Medicine. (1994). *Reducing risks for mental disorders: Frontiers for preventive intervention research.* Washington, DC: National Academy Press.

Price, R. H., Cowen, E. L., Lorion, R. P., & Ramos-McKay, J. (1988).

Fourteen ounces of prevention: A casebook for practitioners. Washington, DC: American Psychological Association.

Roberts, M. C., & Peterson, L. (Eds.). (1984). *Prevention of problems in childhood: Psychological research and applications.* New York: Wiley.

Slavin, R. E., Karweit, N. L., & Wasik, B. A. (Eds.). (1994). *Preventing early school failure: Research, policy and practice.* Needham Heights, MA: Allyn & Bacon.

Slavin, R. E., Karweit, N. L., & Madden, N. A. (Eds.). (1989). *Effective programs for students at risk.* Boston: Allyn & Bacon.

Winett, R. A., King, A. C., & Altman, D. G. (1989). *Health psychology and public health: An integrative approach.* New York: Pergamon.

Since 1975, the University of Vermont has sponsored annual conferences on the primary prevention of psychopathology and published its proceedings. Specific volumes most relevant to prevention for child and adolescent populations are listed chronologically.

Kent, M. W., & Rolf, J. E. (Eds.). (1979). *Social competence in children* (Vol. 3). Hanover, NH: University Press of New England.

Burchard, J. D., & Burchard, S. N. (Eds.). (1987). *Prevention of delinquent behavior* (Vol. 10). Newbury Park, CA: Sage.

Bond, L. A., & Wagner, B. M. (Eds.). (1988). *Families in transition: Primary prevention programs that work* (Vol. 11). Newbury Park, CA: Sage.

Bond, L. A. & Compas, B. E. (Eds.). (1989). *Primary prevention and promotion in the schools* (Vol. 12). Newbury Park, CA: Sage.

Albee, G. W., Bond, L. A. & Monsey, T. V. C. (Eds.). (1992). *Improving children's lives: Global perspectives on prevention* (Vol. 14). Newbury Park, CA: Sage.

COMPUTER RESOURCES

"Prevention Primer" is the reference tool maintained by the US Public Health Service's Center for Substance Use Prevention (CSAP). The site is on the World Wide Web (http://www.health.org/primer/toc.html) and contains information on a variety of prevention-related topics.

The Centers for Disease Control and Prevention operates a home page on the World Wide Web (http://www.cdc.gov.) that offers information on disease prevention and health promotion public health topics.

The Prevention Research Branch of the National Institute of Mental Health sponsors annual conferences on prevention; has an automated fax-on-demand system, Mental Health Fax4U (301) 443-5158; distributes information on prevention (contact Prevention Research Branch at NIMH, 5600 Fishers Lane, Rockville, MD 20857 (phone (301)443-3533); and operates a home page on the World Wide Web (http://www.nimh.gov.)

BIBLIOGRAPHIES

Two extensive bibliographies related to prevention in mental health are recommended:

Buckner, J. C., Trickett, E. J., & Corse, S. J. (1985). *Primary prevention in mental health: An annotated bibliography*. Rockville, MD: DHHS Pub. No. (ADM) 85-1405.

This annotated bibliography contains 1008 published references devoted to primary prevention in mental health appearing through early 1983.

Trickett, E. J., Dahiyat, C., & Selby, P. (1994). *Primary prevention in mental health: An annotated bibliography*, 1983– 1991. Rockville, MD: National Institutes of Health, National Institute of Mental Health (NIH Publication No. 94-3767).

This volume updates the previous bibliography and contains over 1326 publications from 1983 through mid-1991.

JOURNALS

In alphabetical order, the journals most likely to publish articles in prevention include:

American Journal of Community Psychology
American Journal of Public Health
Health Education Quarterly
Journal of Drug Education
Journal of Prevention and Intervention in the Community, (formerly, *Prevention in Human Services*)
Journal of Primary Prevention
Journal of School Health
Preventive Medicine

In addition, examples of special issues or sections of journals that have been devoted to prevention include:

American Journal of Community Psychology. (1982). *10*(3), 235–367, Research in primary prevention in mental health.

American Journal of Community Psychology. (1991). *19*(4), 453–639, Prevention intervention research centers.

American Journal of Community Psychology. (1997). *25*(2), 112–243, Meta-analysis of primary prevention programs.

Journal of Adolescent Research. (1996). *11*(1), 5–163, Preventing adolescent substance abuse.

Journal of Consulting and Clinical Psychology. (1985). *53*(5), 576–646, Primary prevention of childhood disorders.

Journal of Consulting and Clinical Psychology (1995). *53*(4), 515–584, Prediction and prevention of child and adolescent antisocial behavior.

Journal of Social Issues. (1987). *43*(2), 1–167, Children's injuries: Prevention and public policy.

Mental Retardation (1992). *30*(6), 303–369, Prevention of mental retardation and related disabilities.

Preventive Medicine (1996). *25*(4), 377–494, The Multicenter Child and Adolescent Trial for Cardiovascular Health (CATCH): Promoting cardiovascular health through schools.

CLEARINGHOUSES

The Institute of Medicine (1994) (see above) listed 13 clearinghouses in the United States and Canada that provide information related to the prevention of mental disorders. The names, addresses, and phone numbers of these organizations are reproduced below:

1. CSAP National Resource Center for the Prevention of Perinatal Abuse of Alcohol and Other Drugs
   Center for Substance Abuse Prevention
   Substance Abuse and Mental Health Services Administration
   US Department of Health and Human Services
   Lewin-VHI
   9302 Lee Highway
   Suite 310
   Fairfax, VA 32031
   703-218-5600

2. Clearinghouse on Child Abuse and Neglect Information
   National Center on Child Abuse and Neglect
   US Department of Health and Human Services
       PO Box 1182
       Washington, DC 20013-1182
       1-800-FYI-3366
3. Mental Health Policy Resource Center
       1730 Rhode Island Avenue, NW
       Suite 308
       Washington, DC 20036
       202-775-8826
4. National Clearinghouse for Alcohol and Drug Information
   Center for Substance Abuse Prevention
   Substance Abuse and Mental Health Services
   US Department of Health and Human Services
       PO Box 2345
       Rockville, MD 20847-2345
       301-468-2600
5. National Committee to Prevent Child Abuse
       332 South Michigan Avenue
       Suite 1600
       Chicago, IL 60604
       312-663-3520
6. National Criminal Justice Reference Service
   National Institute of Justice Clearinghouse
   Department of Justice
       1600 Research Boulevard
       Dept. F
       Rockville, MD 20850
       1-800-851-3420
7. National Maternal and Child Health Clearinghouse
   Maternal and Child Health Bureau
   US Department of Health and Human Services
       8201 Greensboro Drive - Suite 630
       McLean, VA 22101
       703-821-8955
8. National Mental Health Association
   National Prevention Coalition
       1021 Prince Street
       Alexandria, VA 22314-2971
       703-684-7722

9. National Prevention Evaluation Research Collection
Center for Substance Abuse Prevention
Substance Abuse and Mental Health Services Administration
US Department of Health and Human Services
    Aspen Systems Corporation
    1600 Research Boulevard
    MS-1C
    Rockville, MD 20850
    301-251-5180
10. National Resource Center on Worksite Health Promotion
    777 North Capitol Street, NE
    Suite 800
    Washington, DC 20002
    202-408-9320
11. ODPHP National Health Information Center
Office of Disease Prevention and Health Promotion
US Department of Health and Human Services
    PO Box 1133
    Washington, DC 20013-1133
    1-800-336-4797
12. Ontario Prevention Clearinghouse
The Ministry of Community and Social Services
    415 Yonge Street
    Suite 1200
    Toronto, Ontario M5B 2E7
    Canada
    416-408-2121
13. Resource Center on Substance Abuse Prevention and Disability
    1331 F Street NW
    Suite 800
    Washington, DC 20077-1514
    202-783-2900

OTHER RESOURCES

Franklin, C., Schwab, A. J., Danis, F., Brown, S., & Rattler, L. (1993). A
    review of national school-age pregnancy and prevention informa-
    tion clearinghouses. *Child and Adolescent Social Work Journal, 10,*
    225–239.
These authors provide details on 22 national clearinghouses that
provide information on school-age pregnancy and prevention.

Perry, M. J., Albee, G. W., Bloom, M., & Gullotta, T. P. (1996). Training and career paths in primary prevention. *Journal of Primary Prevention, 16*, 357–371.

Provides information on careers and training in primary prevention available in public health, community psychology, social work and education.

Prevention First Incorporated (PFI), a nonprofit Illinois organization, operates one of the nation's largest prevention libraries, which serves as a clearinghouse for prevention and health promotion activities. PFI operates a lending library and resource center that contains books, videos, training and curriculum manuals, and health education materials. PFI also provides opportunities for information exchange through an electronic bulletin board service. The Web site for PFI is http://www.prevention.org. Contact PFI at (217) 793-7353 (toll free in Illinois at 800-252-8951).

References

Abrahams, N., Casey, K., & Daro, D. (1992). Teachers' knowledge, attitudes, and beliefs about child abuse and its prevention. *Child Abuse and Neglect, 16,* 229–238.

Alan Guttmacher Institute. (1994). *Sex and America's teenagers.* New York: Author.

Allen, J. P., Kuperminc, G., Philliber, S., & Herre, K. (1994). Programmatic prevention of adolescent problem behaviors: The role of autonomy, relatedness, and volunteer service in the Teen Outreach Program. *American Journal of Community Psychology, 22,* 617–638.

Allensworth, D. D. (1993). Health education: State of the art. *Journal of School Health, 63,* 14–20.

Alter-Reid, K., Gibbs, M. S., Lachenmeyer, J. R., Sigal, J., & Massoth, N. A. (1986). Sexual abuse of children: A review of the empirical findings. *Clinical Psychology Review, 6,* 249–266.

American Psychological Association. (1996). *Violence and the family: Report of the American Psychological Association Task Force on Violence and the Family.* Washington, DC: Author.

Arthey, S., & Clarke, V. A. (1995). Suntanning and sun protection: A review of the psychological literature. *Social Science and Medicine, 40,* 265–274.

Backer, T. E., Rogers, E. M., & Sopory, P. (1992). *Designing health communication campaigns: What works?* Newbury Park, CA: Sage.

Baker, S. P. (1981). Childhood injuries: The community approach to prevention. *Journal of Public health Policy, 2,* 235–246.

Ballart, X., & Riba, C. (1995). Impact of legislation requiring moped and motorbike riders to wear helmets. *Evaluation and Program Planning, 18,* 311–320.

Barnett, W. S. (1985). Benefit–cost analysis of the Perry Preschool Program and its policy implications. *Educational Evaluation and Policy Analysis, 7,* 333–342.

Barnett, W. S. (1990). Benefits of compensatory preschool education. *Journal of Human Resources, 27,* 279–312.

Barnett, W. S. (1993). Benefit–cost analysis of preschool education: Findings from a 25-year follow-up. *American Journal of Orthopsychiatry, 63,* 500–508.

Barnett, W. S. (1995). Long-term effects of early childhood programs on cognitive and school outcomes. *Future of Children, 5,* 25–50.

Barnett, W. S., & Escobar, C. M. (1987). The economics of early educational intervention: A review. *Review of Educational Research, 57,* 387–414.

Bass, J. L., Christoffel, K. K., Widome, M., Boyle, W., Scheidt, P., Stanwick, R., & Roberts, K.

(1993). Childhood injury prevention counseling in primary care settings: A critical review of the literature. *Pediatrics, 92,* 544–550.

Becker, W. C., & Carnine, D. W. (1980). Direct Instruction: An effective approach to educational intervention with the disadvantaged and low performers. In B. B. Lahey & A. E. Kazdin (Eds.), *Advances in clinical child psychology, Vol. 3* (pp. 429–473). New York: Plenum.

Becker, W. C., & Gersten, R. (1982). A follow-up of Follow Through: The later effects of the Direct Instruction Model on children in fifth and sixth grades. *American Educational Research Journal, 19,* 75–92.

Beers, C. (1907). *A mind that found itself: An autobiography.* New York: Longmans, Green.

Belsky, J. (1993). Etiology of child maltreatment: A developmental–ecological analysis. *Psychological Bulletin, 114,* 413–434.

Bennett, W. J. (1994). *The index of leading cultural indicators: Facts and figures on the state of American society.* New York: Simon & Schuster.

Bergman, A. B., Rivara, F. P., Richards, D. D., & Rogers, L. W. (1990). The Seattle children's bicycle helmet campaign. *American Journal of Diseases of Children, 144,* 727–731.

Berlin, I. N. (1990). The role of the community mental health center in prevention of infant, child and adolescent disorders: Retrospect and prospect. *Community Mental Health Journal, 26,* 89–106.

Bloch, S. A., & Ungerleider, S. (1988). Whither the drunk driving movement? The social and programmatic orientations of Mothers Against Drunk Driving. *Evaluation and Program Planning, 11,* 237–244.

Boocock, S. S. (1995). Early childhood programs in other nations: Goals and outcomes. *Future of Children, 5,* 94–114.

Botvin, G. J., Baker, E., Dusenbury, L., Botvin, E. M., & Diaz, T. (1995). Long-term follow-up results of a randomized drug abuse prevention trial in a white middle-class population. *Journal of the American Medical Association, 273,* 1106–1112.

Bowen, D. J., Kinne, S., & Orlandi, M. (1995). School policy in COMMIT: A promising strategy to reduce smoking by youth. *Journal of School Health, 65,* 140–144.

Briley, M. E., Roberts-Gray, C., & Rowe, S. (1993). What can children learn from the menu at the child care center? *Journal of Community Health, 18,* 363–377.

Bronfenbrenner, U. (1979). *The ecology of human development: Experiments by nature and design.* Cambridge, MA: Harvard University Press.

Brooks-Gunn, J., Gross, R. T., Kraemer, H. C., Spiker, D., & Shapiro, S. (1992). Enhancing the cognitive outcomes of low birth weight, premature infants: For whom is the intervention most effective? *Pediatrics, 89,* 1209–1215.

Brooks-Gunn, J., McCarton, C. M., Casey, P. H., McCormick, M. C., Bauer, C. R. Bernbaum, J. C., Tyson, J., Swanson, M., Bennett, F. C., Scott, D. T., Tonascia, J., & Meinert, C. L. (1994). Early intervention in low-birth-weight premature infants: Results through age 5 years from the Infant Health and Development Program. *Journal of the American Medical Association, 272,* 1257–1262.

Brooks-Gunn, J., McCormick, M. C., Shapiro, S., Benasich, A. A., & Black, G. W. (1994). The effects of early education intervention on maternal employment, public assistance, and health insurance: The Infant Health and Development Program. *American Journal of Public Health, 84,* 924–931.

Brophy, J. (1986). Teacher influences on student achievement. *American Psychologist, 41,* 1069–1077.

Broussard, E. R. (1982). Primary prevention of psychosocial disorders: Assessment of outcome. In L. A. Bond & J. M. Joffe (Eds.), *Facilitating infant and early childhood development* (pp. 180–196). Hanover, NH: University Press of New England.

Bukstein, O. G. (1995). *Adolescent substance abuse: Assessment, prevention, and treatment*. New York: Wiley.

Campbell, F. A., & Ramey, C. T. (1995). Cognitive and school outcomes for high-risk African-American students at middle adolescence: Positive effects of early intervention. *American Educational Research Journal, 32,* 743–772.

Caplan, G. (1964). *The principles of preventive psychiatry*. New York: Basic Books.

Carnegie Corporation. (1992). *A matter of time: Risk and opportunity in the nonschool hours*. New York: Author.

Carta, J. J. (1992). Education for young children in inner-city classrooms. In T. Thompson & S. C. Hupp (Eds.), *Saving children at risk: Poverty and disabilities* (pp. 71–86). Newbury Park, CA: Sage.

Cartledge, G., & Milburn, J. F. (Eds.). (1980). *Teaching social skills to children: Innovative approaches*. New York: Pergamon.

Chaloupka, F. J., Saffer, H., & Grossman, M. (1993). Alcohol-control policies and motor-vehicle fatalities. *Journal of Legal Studies, 22,* 161–186.

Chamberlin, R. W. (Ed.). (1988). *Beyond individual risk assessment: Communitywide approaches to promoting the health and development of families and children*. Washington, DC: National Center for Education in Maternal and Child Health.

Cheadle, A., Pearson, D., Wagner, E., Psaty, B. M., Diehr, P., & Koepsell, T. (1995). A community-based approach to preventing alcohol use among adolescents on an American Indian reservation. *Public Health Reports, 110,* 439–447.

Cheung, L. W. Y., & Richmond, J. B. (Eds.). (1995). *Child health, nutrition and physical activity*. Champaign, IL: Human Kinetics Press.

Children's Defense Fund. (1995). *The state of America's children yearbook: 1995*. Washington, DC: Author.

Christenson, S. L., Rounds, T., & Gorney, D. (1992). Family factors and student achievement: An avenue to increase students' success. *School Psychology Quarterly, 7,* 178–206.

Christopher, F. S. (1995). Adolescent pregnancy prevention. *Family Relations, 44,* 384–391.

Clarke, G. N., Hawkins, W., Murphy, M., Sheeber, L. B., Lewinsohn, P. M., & Seeley, J. R. (1995). Targeted prevention of unipolar depressive disorder in an at-risk sample of high school adolescents: A randomized trial of a group cognitive intervention. *Journal of the American Academy of Child and Adolescent Psychiatry, 34,* 312–321.

Coben, J. H., Weiss, H. B., Mulvey, E. P., & Dearwater, S. R. (1994). A primer on school violence prevention. *Journal of School Health, 64,* 309–313.

Cohen, D. A., & Linton, K. L. P. (1995). Parent participation in an adolescent drug abuse prevention program. *Journal of Drug Education, 25,* 159–169.

Cohen, P. A., Kulik, J. A., & Kulik, C. C. (1982). Educational outcomes of tutoring: A meta-analysis of findings. *American Educational Research Journal, 19,* 237–248.

Cohn, A. H., & Daro, D. (1987). Is treatment too late? What ten years of evaluative research tell us. *Child Abuse and Neglect, 11,* 433–442.

Coie, J. D., & Krehbiel, G. (1984). Effects of academic tutoring on the social status of low-achieving, socially rejected children. *Child Development, 55,* 1465–1478.

Colan, N. B., Mague, K. C., Cohen, R. S., & Schneider, R. J. (1994). Family education in the workplace: A prevention program for working parents and school-aged children. *Journal of Primary Prevention, 15,* 161–172.

Coleman, J. S. (1972). *Policy research in the social sciences*. Morristown, NJ: General Learning Press.

Collins, J. L., Small, M. L., Kann, L., Pateman, B. C., Gold, R. S., & Kolbe, L. J. (1995). School health education. *Journal of School Health, 65,* 302–311.

Comer, J. P. (1985). The Yale-New Haven Primary Prevention Project: A follow-up study. *Journal of the American Academy of Child and Adolescent Psychiatry, 24,* 154–160.

Compas, B. E., Hinden, R. R., & Gerhardt, C. A. (1995). Adolescent development: Pathways and processes of risk and resilience. *Annual Review of Psychology, 46,* 265–293.

Connell, D. B., Turner, R. R., & Mason, E. F. (1985). Summary of findings of the school health education evaluation: Health promotion effectiveness, implementation, and costs. *Journal of School Health, 55,* 316–321.

Cote, T. R., Sacks, J. J., Lambert-Huber, D. A., Dannenberg, A. L., Kresnow, M. J., Lipsitz, C. M., & Schmidt, E. R. (1992). Bicycle helmet use among Maryland children: Effect of legislation and education. *Pediatrics, 89,* 1216–1220.

Cowen, E. L. (1986). Primary prevention in mental health: Ten years of retrospect and ten years of prospect. In M. Kessler & S. E. Goldston (Eds.), *A decade of progress in primary prevention* (pp. 3–45). Hanover, NH: University Press of New England.

Cowen, E. L. (1994). The enhancement of psychological wellness: Challenges and opportunities. *American Journal of Community Psychology, 22,* 149–180.

Cowen, E. L., Hightower, A. D., Pedro-Carroll, J. P., Work, W. C., & Wyman, P. A. (1996). *School based prevention for children at-risk: The Primary Mental Health Project.* Washington, DC: American Psychological Association.

Crockett, S. J., Mullis, R., Perry, C. L., & Luepker, R. V. (1989). Parent education in youth-directed nutrition interventions. *Preventive Medicine, 18,* 475–491.

Cushman, R., James, W., & Waclawik, H. (1991). Physicians promoting bicycle helmets for children: A randomized trial. *American Journal of Public Health, 81,* 1044–1046.

Dannenberg, A. L., Gielen, A. C., Beilenson, P. L., Wilson, M. H., & Joffe, A. (1993). Bicycle helmet laws and educational campaigns: An evaluation to increase children's helmet use. *American Journal of Public Health, 83,* 667–674.

Davidson, L. L., Durkin, M. S., Kuhn, L., O'Connor, P., Barlow, B., & Heagarty, M. C. (1994). The impact of the Safe Kids/Healthy Neighborhoods Injury Prevention Program in Harlem, 1988 through 1991. *American Journal of Public Health, 84,* 580–586.

DeAngelis, T. (1996, May). How to conduct a successful community-research project. *APA Monitor,* p. 29.

DeCharms, R. (1972). Personal causation training in the schools. *Journal of Applied Social Psychology, 2,* 95–113.

Decker, M. D., Dewey, M. J., Hutcheson, R. H., & Shafner, W. (1984). The use and efficacy of child restraint devices. *Journal of the American Medical Association, 252,* 2571–2575.

Deren, S., Davis, W. R., Tortu, S., Beardsley, M., & Ahluwalia, I. (1995). Women at risk for HIV: Pregnancy and risk behaviors. *Journal of Drug Issues, 27,* 57–71.

Dielman, T. E., Shope, J. T., Leech, S. L., & Butchart, A. T. (1989). Differential effectiveness of an elementary school-based alcohol misuse prevention program. *Journal of School Health, 59,* 255–263.

Digiuseppe, R., & Kassinove, H. (1976). Effects of a rational–emotive school mental health program on children's emotional adjustment. *Journal of Community Psychology, 4,* 382–387.

Dolan, L. J., Kellam, S. G., Hendricks-Brown, C., Werthamer-Larsson, L., Rebok, G. W., Mayer, L. S., Laudolff, J., Turkkan, J. S., Ford, C., & Wheeler, L. (1993). The short-term impact of two classroom-based preventive interventions on aggressive and shy behaviors and poor achievement. *Journal of Applied Developmental Psychology, 14,* 317–345.

Drummond, M., Torrance, G., & Mason, J. (1993). Cost–effectiveness league tables: More harm than good? *Social Science and Medicine, 37,* 33–40.

Dryfoos, J. G. (1990). *Adolescents at risk: Prevalence and prevention*. New York: Oxford University Press.

Dryfoos, J. G. (1995). Full service schools: Revolution or fad? *Journal of Research on Adolescence, 5*, 147–172.

Dunst, C. J., Trivette, C. M., & Thompson, R. B. (1991). Supporting and strengthening family functioning: Toward a congruence between principles and practice. *Prevention in Human Services, 9*, 19–43.

Durlak, J. A. (1977). Description and evaluation of a behaviorally oriented school-based preventive mental health program. *Journal of Consulting and Clinical Psychology, 45*, 27–33.

Durlak, J. A. (1995). *School-based prevention programs for children and adolescents*. Thousand Oaks, CA: Sage.

Durlak, J. A., & Ferrari, J. R. (Eds.). (1993). The importance of program implementation in prevention trials [Special issue]. *Journal of Prevention and Intervention in the Community, 17*(1).

Durlak, J. A., & Gillespie, J. F. (1995). *Assessing the clinical significance of treatment effects in a school-based preventive mental health program*. Unpublished manuscript.

Durlak, J. A., & Wells, A. M. (1997a). Primary prevention mental health programs for children and adolescents: A meta-analytic review. *American Journal of Community Psychology, 25*, 115–152.

Durlak, J. A., & Wells, A. M. (1997b). An evaluation of secondary prevention mental health programs for children and adolescents. *American Journal of Community Psychology*, in press.

Dusenbury, L., Botvin, G. J., & James-Ortiz, S. (1990). The primary prevention of adolescent substance abuse through the promotion of personal and social competence. In R. P. Lorion (Ed.), *Protecting the children: Strategies for optimizing emotional and behavioral development* (pp. 201–224). Binghamton, NY: Haworth.

Elders, M. J., Perry, C. L., Eriksen, M. P., & Giovino, G. A. (1994). The Report of the Surgeon General: Preventing tobacco use among young people. *American Journal of Public Health, 84*, 543–457.

Elias, M. J., Gara, M., & Umbriaco, M. (1985). Sources of stress and support in children's transition to middle school: An empirical analysis. *Journal of Clinical Child Psychology, 14*, 112–118.

Elliott, S. N., & Gresham, F. M. (1993). Social skills interventions for children. *Behavior Modification, 17*, 287–313.

Emery, R. E., & Forehand, R. (1994). Parental divorce and children's well-being: A focus on resilience. In R. J. Haggerty, L. R. Sherrod, N. Garmezy, & M. Rutter (Eds.), *Stress, risk, and resilience in children and adolescents* (pp. 64–99). London, England: Cambridge University Press.

Ennett, S. T., Tobler, N. S., Ringwalt, C. L., & Flewelling, R. L. (1994). How effective is drug abuse resistance education? A meta-analysis of Project DARE outcome evaluations. *American Journal of Public Health, 84*, 1394–1401.

Epstein, J. L. (1990). School and family connections: Theory, research, and implications for integrating sociologies of education and family. *Marriage and Family Review, 15*, 99–126.

Ershoff, D. H., Quinn, V. P., Mullen, P. D., & Lairson, D. R. (1990). Pregnancy and medical cost outcomes of a self-help prenatal smoking cessation program in a HMO. *Public Health Reports, 105*, 340–347.

Evertson, C. M. (1985). Training teachers in classroom management: An experimental in secondary school classrooms. *Journal of Educational Research, 79*, 51–58.

Evertson, C. M., Emmer, E. T., Sanford, J. P., & Clements, B. S. (1983). Improving classroom management: An experiment in elementary school classrooms. *Elementary School Journal, 84,* 173–188.

Falco, M. (1992). *The making of a drug-free America.* New York: Time Books.

Fantuzzo, J. W., King, J. A., & Heller, L. R. (1992). Effects of reciprocal peer tutoring on mathematics and school adjustment: A component analysis. *Journal of Educational Psychology, 84,* 331–339.

Farley, C., Haddad, S., & Brown, B. (1995). The effects of a 4-year program promoting bicycle helmet use among children in Quebec. *American Journal of Public Health, 85,* 46–51.

Fawcett, S. B., Lewis, R. K., Paine-Andrews, A., Francisco, V. T., Richter, K. P., Williams, E. L., & Copple, B. (1996). Evaluating community coalitions for prevention of substance abuse. Manuscript submitted for publication.

Fawcett, S. B., Seekins, T., & Jason, L. A. (1987). Policy research and child passenger safety legislation: A case study and experimental evaluation. *Journal of Social Issues, 43,* 133–148.

Feighery, E., Altman, D. G., & Shaffer, G. (1991). The effects of combining education and enforcement to reduce tobacco sales to minors. *Journal of the American Medical Association, 266,* 3168–3171.

Felner, R. D., Brand, S., Adan, A. M., Mulhall, P. F., Flowers, N., Sartain, B., & DuBois, D. L. (1993). Restructuring the ecology of the school as an approach to prevention during school transitions: Longitudinal follow-ups and extensions of the School Transitional Environment Project (STEP). *Prevention in Human Services, 10,* 103–136.

Felner, R. D., Brand, S., Mulhall, K. E., Counter, B., Millman, J. B., & Fried, J. (1994). The parenting partnership: The evaluation of a human service/corporate workplace collaboration for the prevention of substance abuse and mental health problems, and the promotion of family and work adjustment. *Journal of Primary Prevention, 15,* 123–146.

Fetterman, D., Kafterian, S., & Wandersman, A. (Eds.). (1995). *Empowerment evaluation: Knowledge and tools for self-assessment and accountability.* Thousand Oaks, CA: Sage.

Finkelhor, D., Asdigian, N., & Dziuba-Leatherman, J. (1995a). The effectiveness of victimization prevention instruction: An evaluation of children's responses to actual threats and assaults. *Child Abuse and Neglect, 19,* 141–153.

Finkelhor, D., Asdigian, N., & Dziuba-Leatherman, J. (1995b). Victimization prevention programs for children: A follow-up. *American Journal of Public Health, 85,* 1684–1689.

Finkelhor, D., & Dziuba-Leatherman, J. (1994). Children as victims of violence: A national survey. *Pediatrics, 94,* 413–420.

Finkelhor, D., & Strapko, N. (1992) Sexual abuse prevention education: A review of evaluation studies. In D. J. Willis, E. W. Holden, & M. Rosenberg (Eds.), *Prevention of child maltreatment: Developmental and ecological perspectives* (pp. 150–167). New York: Wiley.

Finney, J. W., Christophersen, E. R., Friman, P. C., Kalnins, I. V., Maddux, J. E., Peterson, L., Roberts, M. C., & Wolraich, M. (1993). Society of Pediatric Psychology Task Force Report: Pediatric psychology and injury control. *Journal of Pediatric Psychology, 18,* 499–526.

Flay, B. R. (1987). *Selling the smokeless society: Fifty-six evaluated mass media programs and campaigns worldwide.* Washington, DC: American Public Health Association.

Floyd, R. L., Rimer, B. K., Giovino, G. A., Mullen, P. D., & Sullivan, S. E. (1993). A review of smoking in pregnancy: Effects on pregnancy outcomes and cessation efforts. *Annual Review of Public Health, 14,* 379–411.

Flynn B. C., & Rains, J. W. (1993). Establishing community coalitions for prevention: Healthy Cities Indiana. In R. N. Knollmueller (Ed.), *Prevention across the life span: Healthy people for the twenty-first century* (pp. 21–30). Washington, DC: American Nurses Publishing.

Flynn, B. S., Worden, J. K., Secker-Walker, R. H., Pirie, P. L., Badger, G. J., Carpenter, J. H., & Geller, B. M. (1994). Mass media and school interventions for cigarette smoking prevention: Effects 2 years after completion. *American Journal of Public Health, 84,* 1148–1150.

Forehand, R., & Long, N. (1988). Outpatient treatment of the acting-out child: Procedures, long-term follow-up data, and clinical problems. *Advances in Behavior Research and Therapy, 10,* 129–177.

Frank, R. G. (1993). Cost–benefit evaluations in mental health: Implications for financing policy. *Advances in Health Economics and Health Services Research, 14,* 1–16.

Fraser, B. J., & Walberg, H. J. (Eds.). (1991). *Educational environments: Evaluation, antecedents and consequences.* New York: Pergamon.

Frazier, F., & Matthes, W. A. (1975). Parent education: A comparison of Adlerian and behavioral approaches. *Elementary School Guidance and Counseling, 10,* 31–38.

Fullan, M. G. (1992). *Successful school improvement*: The implementation perspective and beyond. Philadelphia: Open University Press.

Furstenberg, Jr., F. F., Brooks-Gunn, J., & Morgan, S. P. (1987). *Adolescent mothers in later life.* Cambridge, England: Cambridge University Press.

Gardner, W., & Wilcox, B. L. (1993). Political intervention in scientific peer review: Research on adolescent behavior. *American Psychologist, 48,* 972–983.

Gettinger, M. (1988). Methods of proactive classroom management. *School Psychology Review, 17,* 227–242.

Ginsberg, G. M., & Silverberg, D. S. (1994). A cost–benefit analysis of legislation for bicycle safety helmets in Israel. *American Journal of Public Health, 84,* 653–656.

Girgis, A., Sanson-Fisher, R. W., Tripodi, D. A., & Golding, T. (1993). Evaluation of interventions to improve solar protection in primary schools. *Health Education Quarterly, 20,* 275–287.

Gliksman, L., Allison, K., Adlaf, E., & Newton-Taylor, B. (1995). Toward a comprehensive school drug policy in Ontario. *Journal of Drug Education, 25,* 129–138.

Goldston, S. E. (1986). Primary prevention: Historical perspectives and a blueprint for action. *American Psychologist, 41,* 453–460.

Gramlich, E. (1990). *A guide to benefit–cost analysis.* Englewood Cliffs, NJ: Prentice-Hall.

Greenberg, R. A., Strecher, V. J., Bauman, K. E., Boat, B. W., Fowler, M. G., Keyes, L. L. Denny, F. W., Chapman, R. S., Stedman, H. S., LaVange, L. M., Glover, L. H., Haley, N. J., & Loda, F. A. (1994). Evaluation of a home-based intervention program to reduce infant passive smoking and lower respiratory illness. *Journal of Behavioral Medicine, 17,* 273–290.

Greenwood, C. R., Carta, J. J., & Hall, R. V. (1988). The use of classwide peer tutoring strategies in classroom management and instruction. *School Psychology Review, 17,* 258–275.

Greenwood, C. R., Delquadri, J. C., & Hall, R. V. (1989). Longitudinal effects of classwide peer tutoring. *Journal of Educational Psychology, 81,* 371–383.

Greenwood, C. R., Terry, B., Arreaga-Mayer, C., & Finney, R. (1992). The classwide peer tutoring program: Implementation factors moderating students' achievement. *Journal of Applied Behavior Analysis, 25,* 101–116.

Grossman, M., Chaloupka, F. J., Saffer, H., & Laixuthai, A. (1994). Effects of alcohol price policy on youth: A summary of economic research. *Journal of Research on Adolescence, 4,* 347–364.

Gullotta, T. P. (1994). The what, who, why, where, when, and how of primary prevention. *Journal of Primary Prevention, 15,* 5–14.

Hamblin, R. L., Jacobsen, R. B., & Miller, J. L. L. (1973). *A mathematical theory of social change.* New York: Wiley.

Hansen, W. B., & Graham, J. W. (1991). Preventing alcohol, marijuana, and cigarette use among adolescents: Peer pressure resistance training versus establishing conservative norms. *Preventive Medicine, 20,* 414–430.

Harbeck-Weber, C., & McKee, D. H. (1995). Prevention of emotional and behavioral distress in children experiencing hospitalization and chronic illness. In M. C. Roberts (Ed.), *Handbook of pediatric psychology* (2nd ed., pp. 178–200). New York: Guilford.

Hardy, J. B., & Street, R. (1989). Family support and parenting education in the home: An effective extension of clinic-based preventive health care services for poor children. *Pediatrics, 115,* 927–931.

Hawkins, J. D., Catalano, R. F., & Miller, J. Y. (1992). Risk and protective factors for alcohol and other drug problems in adolescence and early adulthood: Implications for substance abuse prevention. *Psychology Bulletin, 112,* 64–105.

Hawkins, J. D., Von Cleve, E., & Catalano, Jr., H. F. (1991). Reducing early childhood aggression: Results of a primary prevention program. *Journal of the American Academy of Child and Adolescent Psychiatry, 30,* 208–217.

Heller, K., Price, R. H., & Sher, K. J. (1980). Research and evaluation in primary prevention: Issues and guidelines. In R. H. Price, R. F. Ketterer, B. C. Bader, & J. Monahan (Eds.), *Prevention in mental health: Research, policy, and practice* (pp. 285–313). Beverly Hills, CA: Sage.

Henggeler, S. W., Melton, G. B., & Rodrigue, J. R. (1992). *Pediatric and adolescent AIDS: Research findings from the social sciences.* Newbury Park, CA: Sage.

Hetznecker, W., & Forman, M. A. (1971). Community child psychiatry: Evolution and direction. *American Journal of Orthopsychiatry, 41,* 350–370.

Hobfoll, S. E., Jackson, A. P., Lavin, J., Britton, P. J., & Shepherd, J. B. (1994). Reducing inner-city women's AIDS risk activities: A study of single, pregnant women. *Health Psychology, 13,* 397–403.

Horacek, H. J., Ramey, C. T., Campbell, F. A., Hoffmann, K. P., & Fletcher, R. H. (1987). Predicting school failure and assessing early intervention with high-risk children. *Journal of the American Academy of Child and Adolescent Psychiatry, 26,* 758–763.

Horn, M. (1989). *Before it's too late: The child guidance movement in the United States, 1922–1945.* Philadelphia: Temple University Press.

Hu, T., Sung, H., & Keeler, T. E. (1995). Reducing cigarette consumption in California: Tobacco taxes vs. an anti-smoking media campaign. *American Journal of Public Health, 85,* 1218–1222.

Infant Health and Development Program. (1990). Enhancing the outcomes of low-birth-weight, premature infants: A multisite, randomized, trial. *Journal of the American Medical Association, 263,* 3035–3042.

Institute of Medicine. (1988). *The future of public health.* Washington, DC: National Academy Press.

Institute of Medicine. (1994). *Reducing risks for mental disorders: Frontiers for preventive intervention research.* Washington, DC: National Academy Press.

Jason, L. A., Ji, P. Y., Anes, M. D., & Birkhead, S. H. (1991). Active enforcement of cigarette control laws in the prevention of cigarette sales to minors. *Journal of the American Medical Association, 266,* 3159–3161.

Jason, L. A., Johnson, J. H., Danner, K. E., Taylor, S., & Kurasaki, K. S. (1993). A comprehensive, preventive, parent-based intervention for high-risk transfer students. *Prevention in Human Services, 10*, 27–37.

Jason, L. A., Thompson, D., & Rose, T. (1986). Methodological issues in prevention. In B. A. Edelstein & L. Michelson (Eds.), *Handbook of prevention* (pp. 1–19). New York: Plenum.

Jason, L. A., Weine, A. M., Johnson, J. H., Warren-Sohlberg, L., Filippelli, L. A., Turner, E. Y., & Lardon, C. (1992). *Helping transfer students: Strategies for educational and social readjustment.* San Francisco: Jossey-Bass.

Johnson, C. A., Pentz, M. A., Weber, M. D., Dwyer, J. H., Baer, N., MacKinnon, D. P., Hansen, W. B., & Flay, B. R. (1990). Relative effectiveness of comprehensive community programming for drug abuse prevention with high-risk and low-risk adolescents. *Journal of Consulting and Clinical Psychology, 58*, 447–456.

Johnson, D. L. (1988). Primary prevention of behavior problems in young children: The Houston Parent-Child Development Center. In R. H. Price, E. L. Cowen, R. P. Lorion, & J. Ramos-McKay (Eds.), *14 ounces of prevention: A casebook for practitioners* (pp. 44–52). Washington, DC: American Psychological Association.

Johnston, L. D., O'Malley, P. M., & Bachman, J. G. (Eds.). (1995). *National survey results on drug use from The Monitoring the Future Study, 1975–1994. Vol. 1: Secondary school students* (NIH Publication No. 95-4026) Washington, DC: National Institute on Drug Abuse.

Julnes, G., Konefal, M., Pindur, W., & Kim, P. (1994). Community-based perinatal care for disadvantage adolescents: Evaluation of the Resource Mothers Program. *Journal of Community Health, 19*, 41–57.

Jumper, S. A. (1995). A meta-analysis of the relationship of child sexual abuse to adult psychological adjustment. *Child Abuse and Neglect, 19*, 713–728.

Kagitcibasi, C. (1995). Is psychology relevant to global human development issues? Experience from Turkey. *American Psychologist, 50*, 293–300.

Kaiserman, M. J., & Rogers, B. (1991). Tobacco consumption declining faster in Canada than in the US. *American Journal of Public Health, 81*, 902–904.

Kaplan, R. M. (1984). The connection between clinical health promotion and health status. *American Psychologist, 39*, 755–765.

Kaufman, J., & Zigler, E. (1987). Do abused children become abusive parents? *American Journal of Orthopsychiatry, 57*, 186–192.

Kazdin, A. E. (1990). Psychotherapy for children and adolescents. *Annual Review of Psychology, 41*, 21–54.

Kazdin, A. E. (1996). *Conduct disorder in childhood and adolescence* (2nd ed.). Thousand Oaks, CA: Sage.

Kelder, S. H., Perry, C. L., & Klepp, K. I. (1993). Community-wide youth exercise promotion: Long-term outcomes of the Minnesota Heart Health Program and the Class of 1989 study. *Journal of School Health, 63*, 218–223.

Kelder, S. H., Perry, C. L., Lytle, L. A., & Klepp, K. I. (1995). Community-wide youth nutrition education: Long-term outcomes of the Minnesota Heart Health Program. *Health Education Research, Theory and Practice, 10*, 119–131.

Kellam, S. G., Rebok, G. W., Ialongo, N., & Mayer, L. S. (1994). The course and malleability of aggressive behavior from early first grade into middle school: Results of a developmental epidemiologically based preventive trial. *Journal of Child Psychology and Psychiatry, 35*, 259–281.

Kelly, J. A. (1995). Advances in HIV/AIDS education and prevention. *Family Relations, 44*, 345–352.

Kendall-Tackett, K. A., Williams, L. M., & Finkelhor, D. (1993). Impact of sexual abuse on children: A review and synthesis of recent empirical studies. *Psychological Bulletin*, *113*, 164–180.

Kim, S., Williams, C., Coletti, S. D., Hepler, N. & Crutchfield, C. C. (1995). Benefit–cost analysis of drug abuse prevention programs: A macroscopic approach. *Journal of Drug Education*, *25*, 111–127.

King, J. A. (1994). Meeting the needs of at-risk students: A cost analysis of three models. *Educational Evaluation and Policy Analysis*, 16, 1–19.

Kirby, D., Short, L., Collins, J., Rugg, D., Kolbe, L., Howard, L., Miller, B., Sonenstein, F., & Zabin, L. S. (1994). School-based programs to reduce sexual risk behaviors: A review of effectiveness. *Public Health Reports*, *109*, 339–360.

Klein, D. C., & Goldston, S. E. (1977). *Primary prevention: An idea whose time has come.* Department of Health, Education and Welfare Publication No. (ADM) 77-447. Washington, DC: U.S. Government Printing Office.

Klepp, K. I., Kelder, S. H., & Perry, C. L. (1995). Alcohol and marijuana use among adolescents: Long-term outcomes of the Class of 1989 Study. *Annals of Behavioral Medicine*, *17*, 19–24.

Klitzner, M., Gruenewald, P. J., & Bamberger, E. (1990). The assessment of parent-led prevention programs: A preliminary assessment of impact. *Journal of Drug Education*, *20*, 77–94.

Knitzer, J., Steinberg, Z., & Fleisch, B. (1990). *At the schoolhouse door: An examination of programs and policies for children with behavioral and emotional problems.* New York: Bank Street College of Education.

Knoff, H. M., & Batsche, G. M. (1995). Project Achieve: Analyzing a school reform process for at-risk and underachieving students. *School Psychology Review*, *24*, 579–603.

Kohl, J. (1993). School-based child sexual abuse prevention programs. *Journal of Family Violence*, *8*, 137–150.

Kronenfeld, J. J. (1993). *Controversial issues in health care policy.* Newbury Park, CA: Sage.

Ladd, G. W., & Mize, J. (1983). A cognitive–social learning model of social-skill training. *Psychological Review*, *90*, 127–157.

Lamb, H. R., & Zusman, J. (1979). Primary prevention in perspective. *American Journal of Psychiatry*, *136*, 12–17.

Lavelle, J. M., Hovell, M. F., West, M. P., & Walgren, D. R. (1992). Promoting law enforcement for child protection: A community analysis. *Journal of Applied Behavior Analysis*, *25*, 885–892.

Lavigne, J. V., & Faier-Routman, J. (1992). Psychological adjustment to pediatric physical disorders: A meta-analytic review. *Journal of Pediatric Psychology*, *17*, 133–157.

Leigh, B. C., Schafer, J., & Temple, M. T. (1995). Alcohol use and contraception in first sexual experiences. *Journal of Behavioral Medicine*, *18*, 81–95.

Lev, M. A. (1996, July 7). Rise in suicides has Japanese targeting bullies in schoolyards. *The Chicago Tribune*, Section 1, p. 6.

Levine, M., Toro, P. A., & Perkins, D. V. (1993). Social and community interventions. *Annual Review of Psychology*, *44*, 525–558.

Levit, K. R., Lazenby, H. C., Letsch, S. W., & Cowan, C. A. (1991). National health care spending. *Health Affairs*, *10*, 117–130.

Lewit, E. M., & Baker, L. S. (1995). School readiness. *The Future of Children*, *5*, 128–139.

Lipsey, M. W. (1984). Is delinquency prevention a cost–effective strategy? A California perspective. *Journal of Research in Crime and Delinquency*, *21*, 279–302.

Lipsey, M. W., & Wilson, D. B. (1993). The efficacy of psychological, educational and behavioral treatment. *American Psychologist*, *48*, 1181–1209.

Lloyd, J. W., & De Bettencourt, L. U. (1986). Prevention of achievement deficits. In B. A. Edelstein & L. Michelson (Eds.), *Handbook of prevention* (pp. 117–132). New York: Plenum.

Lochman, J. E. (1992). Cognitive–behavioral intervention with aggressive boys: Three-year follow-up and preventive effects. *Journal of Consulting and Clinical Psychology, 60,* 426–432.

Lombard, D., Neubauer, T. E., Canfield, D., & Winett, R. A. (1991). Behavioral community intervention to reduce the risk of skin cancer. *Journal of Applied Behavior Analysis, 24,* 677–686.

Long, B. B. (1989). The Mental Health Association and prevention. In R. C. Hess and J. DeLeon (Eds.), *The National Mental Health Association: Eighty years of involvement in the field of prevention* (pp. 5–44). Binghamton, NY: Haworth.

Lorion, R. P., Caldwell, R. A., & Cowen, E. L. (1976). Effects of a school mental health project: A one-year follow-up. *Journal of School Psychology, 14,* 56–63.

Luepker, R. V., Perry, C. L., McKinlay, S. M., Nader, P. R., Parcel, G. S., Stone, E. J., Webber, L. S., Elder, J. P., Feldman, H. A., Johnson, C. C., Kelder, S. H., & Wu, M. (1996). Outcomes of a field trial to improve children's dietary patterns and physical activity: The Child and Adolescent Trial for Cardiovascular Health (CATCH). *Journal of the American Medical Association, 275,* 768–776.

Lutzker, J. R., & Rice, J. M. (1987). Using recidivism data to evaluate Project 12-Ways: An ecobehavioral approach to the treatment and prevention of child abuse and neglect. *Journal of Family Violence, 2,* 283–290.

Mac Iver, D. J., Reuman, D. A., & Main, S. R. (1995). Social structuring of the school: Studying what is, illuminating what could be. *Annual Review of Psychology, 46,* 375–400.

MacMillan, H. L., MacMillan, J. H., Offord, D. R., Griffith, L., & MacMillan, A. (1994a). Primary prevention of child physical abuse and neglect: A critical review. Part I. *Journal of Child Psychology and Psychiatry, 35,* 835–856.

MacMillan, H. L., MacMillan, J. H., Offord, D. R., Griffith, L., & MacMillan, A. (1994b). Primary prevention of child sexual abuse: A critical review. Part II. *Journal of Child Psychology and Psychiatry, 35,* 857–876.

Malinosky-Rummell, R., & Hansen, D. J. (1993). Long-term consequences of childhood physical abuse. *Psychological Bulletin, 114,* 68–79.

Manning, W. G., Blumberg, L., & Moulton, L. H. (1995). The demand for alcohol: The differential response to price. *Journal of Health Economics, 14,* 123–148.

Manning, W. G., Keeler, E. B., Newhouse, J. P., Sloss, E. M., & Wasserman, J. (1991). *The costs of poor health habits.* Cambridge, MA: Harvard University Press.

Mayer, G. R., & Butterworth, T. W. (1979). A preventive approach to school violence and vandalism: An experimental study. *Personnel and Guidance Journal, 57,* 436–441.

Mayer, G. R., Butterworth, T. W., Nafpaktitis, M., & Sulzer-Azaroff, B. (1983). Preventing school vandalism and improving discipline: A three-year study. *Journal of Applied Behavior Analysis, 16,* 355–369.

McGrath, M. P., & Bogat, G. A. (1995). Motive, intention and authority: Relating developmental research to sexual abuse education for preschoolers. *Journal of Applied Developmental Psychology, 16,* 171–191.

McLeroy, K. R., Bibeau, D., Steckler, A., & Glanz, K. (1988). An ecological perspective on health promotion programs. *Health Education Quarterly, 15,* 351–378.

McMahon, R. J., & Forehand, R. (1984). Parent training for the noncompliant child: Treatment outcome, generalization, and adjunctive therapy procedures. In R. F. Dangel & R. A. Polster (Eds.), *Parent training: Foundations of research and practice* (pp. 298–328). New York: Guilford.

Mechanic, D. (1989). *Mental health and social policy* (3rd ed.). Englewood Cliffs, NJ: Prentice-Hall.

Meehan, M. P., Durlak, J. A., & Bryant, F. B. (1993). The relationship of social support to perceived control and subjective mental health in adolescents. *Journal of Community Psychology, 21*, 49–55.

Melamed, B.G., & Siegel, L. J. (1975). Reduction of anxiety in children facing hospitalization and surgery by use of filmed modeling. *Journal of Consulting and Clinical Psychology, 43*, 511–521.

Melton, G. B. (1992). The improbability of prevention of sexual abuse. In D. J. Willis, E. W. Holden, & M. Rosenberg (Eds.), *Prevention of child maltreatment: Developmental and ecological perspectives* (pp. 169–189). New York: Wiley.

Meyer, L. A. (1984). Long-term academic effects of the direct instruction project: Project Follow Through. *Elementary School Journal, 84*, 380–394.

Miller, T. R., & Galbraith, M. (1995). Injury prevention counseling by pediatricians: A benefit–cost comparison. *Pediatrics, 96*, 1–4.

Morrison, F. J., Griffith, E. M., Williamson, G., & Hardway, C. L. (1995). *The nature and sources of early literacy.* Paper presented at the Society for Research in Child Development, Indianapolis, IN.

Morrow, R. H., & Bryant, J. H. (1995). Health policy approaches to measuring and valuing human life: Conceptual and ethical issues. *American Journal of Public Health, 85*, 1356–1360.

Moser, Jr., R., McCance, K. L., & Smith, K. R. (1991). Results of a national survey of physicians knowledge and application of prevention capabilities. *American Journal of Preventive Medicine, 7*, 384–390.

Murphy, J. (Ed.). (1990). *The educational reform movement of the 1980s.* Berkeley, CA: McCutchan.

National Academy of Sciences. (1985). *Injury to America: A continuing public health problem.* Washington, DC: National Academy Press.

National Commission on Children. (1991). *Beyond rhetoric: A new American agenda for children and families.* Washington, DC: US Government Printing Office.

National Committee for Injury Prevention and Control. (1989). *Injury prevention: Meeting the challenge.* New York: Oxford University Press.

National Institute of Education. (1978). *The safe school study.* Washington, DC: US Department of Health, Education, and Welfare, Office of Education.

National Safety Council. (1993). *Accident facts, 1993 ed.* Itasca, IL: Author.

Nolin, M. J., Davies, E., & Chandler, K. (1996). Student victimization at school. *Journal of School Health, 66*, 216–221.

Nottelmann, E. D., & Jensen, P. S. (1995). Comorbidity of disorders in children and adolescents: Developmental perspectives. In T. H. Ollendick & R. J. Prinz (Eds.), *Advances in clinical child psychology*, (Vol. 17, pp. 109–156). New York: Plenum.

Oakland, T. (1994). Issues of importance to the membership of the American Psychological Association. *American Psychologist, 49*, 879–886.

Oates, R. K., & Bross, D. C. (1995). What have we learned about treating child physical abuse: A literature review of the last decade. *Child Abuse & Neglect, 19*, 463–473.

Oden, S., & Asher, S. R. (1977). Coaching children in social skills for friendship making. *Child Development, 48*, 495–506.

O'Donnell, J., Hawkins, J. D., Catalano, R. F., Abbott, R. D., & Day, L. E. (1995). Preventing school failure, drug use, and delinquency among low-income children: Effects of a long-term prevention project in elementary schools. *American Journal of Orthopsychiatry, 65*, 87–100.

Office of the Inspector General. (1990). *Youth access to cigarettes.* Washington, DC: US Department of Health and Human Services.

Ojemann, R. H., Levitt, E. E., Lyle, W. H., & Whiteside, M. F. (1955). The effects of a "causal" teacher-training program and certain curricular changes on grade school children. *Journal of Experimental Education, 24*, 95–114.

Olds, D. L., Henderson, Jr., C. R., Chamberlin, R., & Tatelbaum, R. (1986). Preventing child abuse and neglect: A randomized trial of nurse home visitation. *Pediatrics, 78*, 65–78.

Olds, D. L., Henderson, C. R., Phelps, C., Kitzman, H., & Hanks, C. (1993). Effect of prenatal and infancy nurse home visitation on government spending. *Medical Care, 31*, 155–174.

Olds, D. L., Henderson, C. R., & Kitzman, H. (1994). Does prenatal and infancy nurse home visitation have enduring effects on qualities of parental caregiving and child health at 25 to 50 months of life? *Pediatrics, 93*, 89–98.

Olds, D. L., & Kitzman, H. (1993). Review of research on home visiting for pregnant women and parents of young children. *The Future of Children, 3*, 53–92.

Olweus, D. (1994). Bullying at school: Basic facts and effects of a school-based intervention program. *Journal of Child Psychology and Psychiatry, 35*, 1171–1190.

O'Malley, P. M., & Wagenaar, A. C. (1991). Effects of minimum drinking age laws on alcohol use, related behaviors and traffic crash involvement among American youth: 1976–1987. *Journal of Studies on Alcohol, 52*, 568–579.

O'Sullivan, A. L., & Jacobsen, B. S. (1992). A randomized trial of a health care program for first-time adolescent mothers and their infants. *Nursing Research, 41*, 210–215.

Palumbo, D. J., & Calista, D. J. (Eds.). (1990). *Implementation and the policy process: Opening up the black box.* New York: Greenwood Press.

Pedro-Carroll, J. L., & Cowen, E. L. (1985). The Children of Divorce Intervention Program: An investigation of the efficacy of a school-based prevention program. *Journal of Consulting and Clinical Psychology, 53*, 603–611.

Pentz, M. A., Brannon, B. R., Charlin, V. L., Barrett, E. J., MacKinnon, D. P., & Flay, B. R. (1989). The power of policy: The relationship of smoking policy to adolescent smoking. *American Journal of Public Health, 79*, 857–862.

Pendergrast, R. A., Ashworth, C. S., DuRant, R. H., & Litaker, M. (1992). Correlates of children's bicycle helmet use and short-term failure of school-level interventions. *Pediatrics, 90*, 354–358.

Perry, C. L., Crockett, S. J., & Pirie, P. (1987). Influencing parental health behavior: Implications of community assessments. *Health Education, 18*, 68–77.

Perry, C. L., Luepker, R. V., Murray, D. M., Kurth, C., Mullis, R., Crockett, S., & Jacobs, Jr., D. R. (1988). Parent involvement with children's health promotion: The Minnesota Home Team. *American Journal of Public Health, 78*, 1156–1160.

Perry, C. L., Murray, D. M., & Griffin, G. (1990). Evaluating the statewide dissemination of smoking prevention curricula: Factors in teacher compliance. *Journal of School Health, 60*, 501–504.

Perry, C. L., Kelder, S. H., Murray, D. M., & Klepp, K. I. (1992). Community-wide smoking prevention: Long-term outcomes of the Minnesota Heart Health Program. *American Journal of Public Health, 82*, 1210–1216.

Perry, C. L., Williams, C. L., Veblen-Mortenson, S., Toomey, T. L., Komro, K. A., Anstine, P. S., McGovern, P. G., Finnegan, J. R., Forster, J. L., Wagenaar, A. C., & Wolfson, M. (1996). Project Northland: Outcomes of a community-wide alcohol use prevention program during early adolescence. *American Journal of Public Health, 86*, 956–965.

Peterson, D. E., Zeger, S. L., Remington, P. L., & Anderson, H. A. (1992). The effect of state cigarette tax increases on cigarette sales, 1955 to 1988. *American Journal of Public Health, 82,* 94–96.

Peterson, L. (1989). Latchkey children's preparation for self-care: Overestimated, under-rehearsed and unsafe. *Journal of Clinical Child Psychology, 18,* 36–43.

Peterson, L., & Brown, D. (1994). Integrating child injury and abuse-neglect research: Common histories, etiologies and solutions. *Psychological Bulletin, 116,* 293–315.

Peterson, L., & Roberts, M. C. (1992). Complacency, misdirection, and effective prevention of children's injuries. *American Psychologist, 23,* 375–387.

Peterson, L., Schultheis, K., Rildey-Johnson, R., Miller, D. J., & Tracy, K. (1984). Comparison of three modeling procedures on the presurgical and postsurgical reactions of children. *Behavior Therapy, 15,* 197–203.

Peterson, L., Mori, L., Selby, V., & Rosen, B. N. (1988). Community interventions in children's injury prevention: Differing costs and differing benefits. *Journal of Community Psychology, 16,* 188–204.

Philliber, S., & Allen, J. P. (1992). Life options and community service: Teen Outreach Program. In B. C. Miller, J. J. Card, R. L. Paikoff, & J. L. Peterson (Eds.), *Preventing adolescent pregnancy: Model programs and evaluations* (pp. 139–155). Newbury Park, CA: Sage.

Pless, I. B., & Arsenault, L. (1987). The role of health education in the prevention of injuries to children. *Journal of Social Issues, 43,* 87–104.

Preusser, D. F., & Williams, A. F. (1992). Sales of alcohol to underage purchasers in three New York countries and Washington, DC. *Journal of Public Health Policy, 13,* 306–317.

Price, R. H. (1986). Education for prevention. In M. Kessler & S. E. Goldston (Eds.), *A decade of progress in primary prevention* (pp. 289–306). Hanover, NH: University Press of New England.

Ramey, C. T., Bryant, D. M., Wasik, B. H., Sparling, J. J., Fendt, K. H., & LaVange, L. M. (1992). Infant Health and Development Program for low birth weight, premature infants: Program elements, family participation, and child intelligence. *Pediatrics, 89,* 454–465.

Randolph, M. K., & Gold, C. A. (1994). Child sexual abuse prevention: Evaluation of a teacher training program. *School Psychology Review, 23,* 485–495.

Reppucci, N. D., & Haugaard, J. J. (1989). Prevention of child sexual abuse: Myth or reality. *American Psychologist, 44,* 1266–1275.

Resnicow, K., Cohn, L., Reinhardt, J., Cross, D., Futterman, R., Kirschner, E., Wynder, E. L., & Allegrante, J. P. (1992). A three-year evaluation of the Know Your Body Program in inner-city schoolchildren. *Health Education Quarterly, 19,* 463–480.

Rice, D. P., & LaPlante, M. P. (1992). Medical expenditures for disability and disabling comorbidity. *American Journal of Public Health, 82,* 739–741.

Richardson, T. R. (1989). *The century of the child: The mental hygiene movement and social policy in the United States and Canada.* Albany: State University of New York Press.

Rickel, A. U., & Lampi, L. (1981). A two-year follow-up study of a preventive mental health program for preschoolers. *American Journal of Community Psychology, 9,* 455–464.

Rickel, A. U., Smith, R. L., & Sharp, K. C. (1979). Description and evaluation of a preventive mental health program for preschoolers. *Journal of Abnormal Child Psychology, 7,* 101–112.

Riessman, F. (1965). The helper therapy principle. *Social Work, 10,* 27–32.

Rigotti, N. A., & Pashos, C. L. (1991). No-smoking laws in the United States: An analysis of state and city actions to limit smoking in public places and workplaces. *Journal of the American Medical Association, 266,* 3162–3167.

Rivara, F. P., & Mueller, B. A. (1987). The epidemiology and causes of childhood injuries. *Journal of Social Issues, 43*, 13–21.

Roberts, M. C. (1987). Public health and health psychology: Two cats of Kilkenny? *Professional Psychology: Research and Practice, 18*, 145–149.

Roberts, M. C., Fanurik, D., & Layfield, D. A. (1987). Behavioral approaches to prevention of childhood injuries. *Journal of Social Issues, 43*, 105–118.

Roberts, M. C., Fanurik, D., & Wilson, D. R. (1988). A community program to reward children's use of seat belts. *American Journal of Community Psychology, 16*, 395–407.

Roberts, M. C., Layfield, D. A., & Fanurik, D. (1992). Motivating children's use of car safety devices. *Advances in Developmental and Behavioral Pediatrics, 10*, 61–88.

Roberts, M. C., & Turner, D. S. (1984). Preventing death and injury in childhood: A synthesis of child safety seat efforts. *Health Education Quarterly, 11*, 181–193.

Robertson, L. S. (1983). *Injuries: Causes, control strategies, and public policy.* Lexington, MA: Lexington Books.

Rodriguez, J. G. (1990). Childhood injuries in the United States: A priority issue. *American Journal of Diseases of Children, 144*, 625–626.

Rogers, M. M., Peoples-Sheps, M. D., & Sorenson, J. R. (1995). Translating research into MCH service: Comparison of a pilot project and a large-scale resource mothers program. *Public Health Reports, 110*, 563–569.

Ross, G. R. (1978). Reducing irrational personality traits, trait anxiety, and intra-interpersonal needs in high school students. *Measurement and Evaluation in Guidance, 11*, 44–49.

Ross, J. G., Einhaus, K. E., Hohenemser, L. K., Greene, B. Z., Kann, L., & Gold, R. S. (1995). School health policies prohibiting tobacco use, alcohol and other drug use, and violence. *Journal of School Health, 65*, 333–338.

Ross, S., & Kantor, L. M. (1995). Trends in opposition to comprehensive sexuality education in public schools: 1994–1995 school year. *Siecus Report, 23*, 9–15.

Rotheram-Borus, M. J., Koopman, C., Haignere, C., & Davies, M. (1991). Reducing HIV sexual risk behaviors among runaway adolescents. *Journal of the American Medical Association, 266*, 1237–1241.

Rowan, B., & Guthrie, L. F. (1989). The quality of Chapter 1 instruction: Results from a study of twenty-four schools. In R. Slavin, N. L. Karweit, & N. A. Madden (Eds.), *Effective programs for students at risk* (pp. 195–219). Needham Heights, MA: Allyn & Bacon.

Russell, L. B. (1986). *Is prevention better than cure?* Washington, DC: The Brookings Institution.

Rutter, M. (1979). Protective factors in children's responses to stress and disadvantage. In M. Whalen & J. E. Rolf (Eds.), *Primary prevention of psychopathology: Vol. 3. Social Competence in Children* (pp. 49–74). Hanover, NH: University Press of New England.

Sameroff, A. J. (1987). Transactional risk factors and prevention. In J. A. Steinberg & M. M. Silverman (Eds.), *Preventing mental disorders: A research perspective* (pp. 74–89). Rockville, MD: National Institute of Mental Health.

Sameroff, A. J., Seifer, R., Zax, M., & Barocas, R. (1987). Early indicators of developmental risk: The Rochester Longitudinal Study. *Schizophrenia Bulletin, 13*, 383–394.

Samet, J. M., Lewit, E. M., & Warner, K. E. (1994). Involuntary smoking and children's health. *The Future of Children, 4*, 94–113.

Sandler, I. N. (Ed.). (1997). Meta-analysis of primary prevention programs. [Special issue] *American Journal of Community Psychology, 25*(2), 112–243.

Sarason, S. B. (1993). *The case for change: Rethinking the preparation of educators.* San Francisco: Jossey-Bass.

Schelp, L. (1987). Community intervention and changes in accident pattern in a rural Swedish municipality. *Health Promotion, 2,* 109–125.

Schelp, L. (1988). The role of organizations in community participation: Prevention of accidental injuries in a rural Swedish municipality. *Social Science and Medicine, 26,* 1087–1093.

Schinke, S. P. (1994). Prevention science and practice: An agenda for action. *Journal of Primary Prevention, 15,* 45–57.

Schinke, S. P., Botvin, G. J., & Orlandi, M. A. (1991). *Substance abuse in children and adolescents: Evaluation and intervention.* Newbury Park, CA: Sage.

Schwartz, D. F., Grisso, J. A., Miles, C., Holmes, J. H., & Sutton, R. L. (1993). An injury prevention program in an urban African-American community. *American Journal of Public Health, 83,* 675–680.

Schweinhart, L. J., & Weikart, D. B. (1988). The High/Scope Perry Preschool Program. In R. H. Price, E. L. Cowen, R. P. Lorion, & J. Ramos-McKay (Eds.), *14 ounces of prevention: A casebook for practitioners* (pp. 53–65). Washington, DC: American Psychological Association.

Seekins, T., Fawcett, S. B., Cohen, S. H., Elder, J. P., Jason, L. A., Schnelle, J. F., & Winett, R. A. (1988). Experimental evaluation of public policy: The case of state legislation for passenger safety. *Journal of Applied Behavior Analysis, 21,* 233–243.

Simmons, S. J. (1993). The economics of prevention. In R. N. Knollmueller, (Ed.). (1993). *Prevention across the life span: Healthy people for the twenty-first century* (pp. 1–9). Washington, DC: American Nurses Publishing.

Simons-Morton, B. G., Parcel, G. S., Baranowski, T., Forthofer, R., & O'Mara, N. M. (1991). Promoting physical activity and a healthful diet among children: Results of a school-based intervention study. *American Journal of Public Health, 81,* 986–991.

Simons-Morton, B. G., Parcel, G. S., & O'Mara, N. M. (1988). Implementing organizational changes to promote healthful diet and physical activity at school. *Health Education Quarterly, 15,* 115–130.

Simons-Morton, B. G., Taylor, W. C., Snider, S. A., & Huang, I. W. (1993). The physical activity of fifth-grade students during physical education classes. *American Journal of Public Health, 83,* 262–264.

Skretny, M. T., Cummings, M., Sciandra, R., & Marshall, J. (1990). An intervention to reduce the sale of cigarettes to minors. *New York State Journal of Medicine, 90,* 54–55.

Slavin, R. E., Karweit, N. L., & Madden, N. A. (1989). *Effective programs for students at risk.* Needham Heights, MA: Allyn & Bacon.

Slavin, R. E., Karweit, N. L., & Wasik, B. A. (1994). *Preventing early school failure.* Needham Heights, MA: Allyn & Bacon.

Smith, G. S., & Falk, H. (1987). Unintentional injuries. In R. W. Ambler & N. B. Dold (Eds.), *Closing the gap: The burden of unnecessary illness* (pp. 143–163). New York: Oxford University Press.

Snortum, J. R. (1988). On seeing the forest and the trees: The need for contextual analysis in evaluating drunk driving policies. *Evaluation and Program Planning, 11,* 279–294.

Soriano, M., Soriano, F. I., & Jimenez, E. (1994). School violence among culturally diverse populations: Sociocultural and institutional considerations. *School Psychology Review, 23,* 216–235.

Spaulding, J., & Balch, P. (1983). A brief history of primary prevention in the twentieth century: 1908 to 1980. *American Journal of Community Psychology, 11,* 59–80.

Spiegel, C. N., & Lindaman, F. C. (1977). Children Can't Fly: A program to prevent childhood morbidity and mortality from window falls. *American Journal of Public Health, 67,* 1143–1147.

Spivack, G., & Shure, M. (1974). *Social adjustment of young children: A cognitive approach to solving real-life problems.* San Francisco: Jossey Bass.

Stephens, T. M. (1978). *Social skills in the classroom.* Columbus, OH: Cedars Press.

Stevens, R. J., & Slavin, R. E. (1995). The cooperative elementary school: Effects on students' achievement, attitudes, and social relations. *American Educational Research Journal, 32,* 321–351.

Stevenson, H. W., Chen, C., & Lee, S. (1993). Mathematics achievement of Chinese, Japanese, and American children: Ten years later. *Science, 259,* 53–58.

St. Lawrence, J. S., Brasfield, T. L., Shirley, A., Jefferson, K. W., Alleyne, E., & O'Bannon, III, R. E. (1995). Cognitive–behavioral intervention to reduce African American adolescents risk for HIV infection. *Journal of Consulting and Clinical Psychology, 63,* 221–237.

Stolberg, A. L., & Mahler, J. (1994). Enhancing treatment gains in a school-based intervention for children of divorce through skill training, parental involvement, and transfer procedures. *Journal of Consulting and Clinical Psychology, 62,* 147–156.

St. Pierre, T. L., Kaltreider, L., Mark, M. N., & Aiken, K. J. (1992). Drug prevention in a community setting: A longitudinal study of the relative effectiveness of a three-year primary prevention program in Boys and Girls Clubs across the nation. *American Journal of Community Psychology, 20,* 673–706.

Sylva, K. (1994). School influences on children's development. *Journal of Child Psychology and Psychiatry, 35,* 135–170.

Tengs, T. O., Adams, M. E., Pliskin, J. S., Safran, D. G., Siegel, J. E., Weinstein, M. C., & Graham, J. D. (1994). Five-hundred life-saving interventions and their cost-effectiveness. *Manuscript submitted for publication.*

Terman, D. L., Larner, M. B., Stevenson, C. S., & Behrman, R. E. (1996). Special education for students with disabilities: Analysis and recommendations. *The Future of Children, 6,* 4–24.

Thompson, R. S., Thompson, D. C., Rivara, F. P., & Salazar, A. A. (1993). Cost-effectiveness analysis of bicycle helmet subsidies in a defined population. *Pediatrics, 91,* 902–907.

Tremblay, R. E., Pagani-Kurtz, L., Masse, L. C., Vitaro, F., & Pihl, R. O. (1995). A bimodal preventive intervention for disruptive kindergarten boys: Its impact through mid-adolescence. *Journal of Consulting and Clinical Psychology, 63,* 560–568.

Tremblay, R. E., Vitaro, F., Bertrand, L., LeBlanc, M., Beauchesne, H., Boileau, H., & David, L. (1992). Parent and child training to prevent early onset of delinquency: The Montreal longitudinal-experimental study. In J. McCord & R. E. Tremblay (Eds.), *Preventing antisocial behavior: Interventions from birth through adolescence* (pp. 117–137). New York: Guilford.

Tyack, D. (1992). Health and social services in public schools: Historical perspectives. *The Future of Children, 2,* 19–31.

United States Department of Education. (1992). *The condition of education, 1992.* Washington, DC: US Department of Education, National Center for Education Statistics.

United States Department of Health and Human Services. (1990). *The health benefits of smoking cessation.* US Department of Health and Human Services, Public Health Service, Centers for Disease Control, Center for Chronic Disease Prevention and Health Promotion, Office on Smoking and Health. DHHS Publication No. (CDC) 90-8416.

United States Preventive Services Task Force. (1989). *Guide to clinical preventive services: An assessment of 169 interventions.* Baltimore: Williams and Wilkins.

van den Boom, D. C. (1995). Do first-year intervention effects endure? Follow-up during toddlerhood of a sample of Dutch irritable infants. *Child Development, 66,* 1798–1816.

Vartiainen, E., Pallonen, U., McAlister, A. L., & Puska, P. (1990). Eight-year follow-up results of an adolescent smoking prevention program: The North Karelia Youth Project. *American Journal of Public Health, 80*, 78–79.

Vaux, A. (1988). *Social support: Theory, research, and intervention.* New York: Praeger.

Vegega, M. E., & Klitzner, M. D. (1988). What have we learned about youth anti-drinking–driving programs? *Evaluation and Program Planning, 11*, 203–217.

Wagenaar, A. C., & Wolfson, M. (1994). Enforcement of the legal minimum drinking age in the United States. *Journal of Public Health Policy, 16*, 37–53.

Wagenaar, A. C., & Wolfson, M. (1995). Deterring sales and provision of alcohol to minors: A study of enforcement in 295 counties in four states. *Public health Reports, 110*, 419–427.

Walberg, H. J. (1984). Improving the productivity of America's schools. *Educational Leadership, 41*, 19–30.

Wall, M. A., Severson, H. H., Andrews, J. A. Lichtenstein, E., & Zoref, L. (1995). Pediatric office-based smoking intervention: Impact on maternal smoking and relapse. *Pediatrics, 96*, 622–628.

Wallack, L., Dorfman, L., Jernigan, D., & Themba, M. (1993). *Media advocacy and public health: Power for prevention.* Newbury Park, CA: Sage.

Walton, W. W. (1982). An evaluation of the poison prevention packaging act. *Pediatrics, 69*, 363–370.

Wasserman, J., Manning, W. G., Newhouse, J. P., & Winkler, J. D. (1991). The effects of excise taxes and regulations on cigarette smoking. *Journal of Health Economics, 10*, 43–64.

Weisbrod, B. A., Test, M. A., & Stein, L. I. (1980). Alternative to mental hospital treatment. *Archives of General Psychiatry, 37*, 400–405.

Weisz, J. R., Weiss, B., Han, S. S., Granger, D. A., & Morton, T. (1995). Effects of psychotherapy with children and adolescents revisited; A meta-analysis of treatment outcome studies. *Psychological Bulletin, 117*, 450–468.

Wesch, D., & Lutzker, J. R. (1991). A comprehensive 5-year evaluation of Project 12-Ways: An eco-behavioral program for treating and preventing child abuse and neglect. *Journal of Family Violence, 6*, 17–35.

Widom, C. S. (1989). Does violence beget violence? A critical examination. *Psychological Bulletin, 106*, 3–28.

Williams, A. F., Rich, R. F., Zador, P. L., & Robertson, L. S. (1975). The legal minimum drinking age and fatal motor vehicle crashes. *Journal of Legal Studies, 4*, 219–239.

Williams, S., Anderson, J., McGee, R., & Silva, P. A. (1990). Risk factors for behavioral and emotional disorder in preadolescent children. *Journal of the American Academy of Child and Adolescent Psychiatry, 29*, 413–419.

Willis, D. J., Holden, E. W., & Rosenberg, M. (Eds.). (1992). Prevention of child maltreatment: Developmental and ecological perspectives. New York: Wiley.

Wilson, M. H., Baker, S. P., Teret, S. P., Shock, S., Garbarino, J. (1991). *Saving children: A guide to injury prevention.* New York: Oxford University Press.

Windsor, R. A., Lowe, J. B., Perkins, L. L., Smith-Yoder, D., Artz, L., Crawford, M., Amburgy, K., & Boyd, N. R. (1993). Health education for pregnant smokers: Its behavioral impact and cost benefit. *American Journal of Public Health, 83*, 201–206.

Winett, R. A., & Anderson, E. S. (1994). HIV prevention in youth: A framework for research and action. In T. H. Ollendick & R. J. Prinz (Eds.), *Advances in clinical child psychology* (Vol. 16, pp. 1–43). New York: Plenum.

Wolf, M. M. (1978). Social validity: The case for subjective measurement, or how behavior analysis is finding its heart. *Journal of Applied Behavior Analysis, 11*, 203–214.

Wolfe, D. A., Reppucci, N. D., & Hart, S. (1995). Child abuse prevention: Knowledge and priorities. *Journal of Clinical Child Psychology, 24*(Suppl.), 5–22.

Wolfe, D. A., & Wekerle, C. (1993). Treatment strategies for child physical abuse and neglect: A critical progress report. *Clinical Psychology Review, 13,* 473–500.

Wolfson, M., Wagenaar, A. C., & Hornseth, G. W. (1995). Law officers' views on enforcement of the minimum drinking age: A four-state study. *Public Health Reports, 110,* 428–438.

Wood, T., & Milne, P. (1988). Head injuries to pedal cyclists and the promotion of helmet use in Victoria, Australia. *Accident Annals of Prevention, 20,* 177–185.

Writing Group for the DISC Collaborative Research Group. (1995). Efficacy and safety of lowering dietary intake of fat and cholesterol in children with elevated low-density lipoprotein cholesterol: The Dietary Intervention Study in Children (DISC). *Journal of the American Medical Association, 273,* 1429–1435.

Yap, J. N. (1988). The effects of hospitalization and surgery on children: A critical review. *Journal of Applied Developmental Psychology, 9,* 349–358.

Yates, B. T. (1985). Cost–effectiveness analysis and cost-benefit analysis: An introduction. *Behavioral Assessment, 7,* 207–234.

Yeaton, W. H., & Bailey, J. S. (1983). Utilization analysis of a pedestrian safety training program. *Journal of Applied Behavior Analysis, 16,* 203–216.

Yoshikawa, H. (1995). Long-term effects of early childhood programs on social outcomes and delinquency. *The Future of Children, 5,* 51–75.

Zabin, L. S., Hirsch, M. B., Street, R., Emerson, M. R., Hardy, J. B., & King, T. M. (1986). The Baltimore Pregnancy Prevention Program for urban teenagers. I. How did it work? *Family Planning Perspectives, 20,* 182–187.

Zimmerman, S. L. (1995). *Understanding family policy: Theories and applications* (2nd ed.). Thousand Oaks, CA: Sage.

Zingraff, M. T., Leiter, J., Johnsen, M. C. & Myers, K. A. (1994). The mediating effect of good school performance on the maltreatment–delinquency relationship. *Journal of Research in Crime and Delinquency, 31,* 62–91.

Author Index

Abrahams, N., 140, 213
Alan Guttmacher Institute, 107, 213
Albee, G. W., 206
Allen, J. P., 109, 111, 112, 178, 179, 213
Allensworth, D. D., 189, 213
Alter-Reid, K., 132, 213
American Psychological Association, 27, 136, 213
Arthey, S., 101, 213

Backer, T. E., 197, 213
Baker, S. P., 118, 213
Ballart, X., 191, 213
Barnett, W. S., 58, 59, 143, 144, 147, 148, 178, 179, 180, 186, 213
Bass, J. L., 129, 200, 213
Becker, W. C., 66, 214
Belsky, J., 133, 214
Bennett, W. J., 28, 214
Bergman, A. B., 121, 122, 214
Berlin, I. N., 20, 214
Bloch, S. A., 174, 214
Bloom, M., 205
Bond, L. A., 206
Boocock, S. S., 59, 61, 214
Botvin, G. J., 77, 78, 214
Bowen, D. J., 161, 214
Briley, M. E., 105, 214

Bronfenbrenner, U., 4, 214
Brooks-Gunn, J., 93, 214
Brophy, J., 67, 214
Broussard, E. R., 32, 214
Bukstein, O. G., 76, 215
Buckner, J. C., 207
Burchard, J. D., 206

Campbell, F. A., 60, 61, 178, 215
Caplan, G., 1, 215
Carnegie Corporation, 195, 215
Carta, J. J., 174, 215
Cartledge, G., 204
Chaloupka, F. J., 164, 167, 215
Chamberlin, R. W., 95, 215
Cheadle, A., 77, 78, 82, 85, 215
Cheung, L. W. Y., 98, 215
Children's Defense Fund, 57, 87, 105, 131, 136, 215
Christenson, S. L., 70, 215
Christopher, F. S., 107, 112
Clarke, G. N., 44, 45, 51, 178, 179, 215
Coben, J. H., 28, 215
Cohen, D. A., 42, 215
Cohen, P. A., 63, 215
Cohn, A. H., 132, 215
Coie, J. D., 73, 215
Colan, N. B., 42, 195, 215
Coleman, J. S., 173, 215

Collins, J. L., 21, 215
Comer, J. P., 73, 75, 216
Compas, B. E., 14, 17, 216
Connell, D. B., 99, 100, 216
Cote, T. R., 121, 122, 216
Cowen, E. L., 2, 13, 45, 73, 205, 216
Crockett, S. J., 102, 216
Cushman, R., 122, 216

Dannenberg, A. L., 121, 216
Davidson, L. L., 124, 125, 216
DeAngelis, T., 197, 216
DeCharms, R., 31, 216
Decker, M. D., 118, 216
Deren, S., 110, 216
Dielman, T. E., 78, 216
Digiuseppe, R., 31, 216
Dolan, L. J., 30, 31, 216
Drummond, M., 146, 216
Dryfoos, J. G., 55, 112, 205, 217
Dunst, C. J., 95, 217
Durlak, J. A., vii, 7, 28, 29, 35, 41, 43, 45, 46, 47, 49, 60, 175, 180, 186, 193, 194, 205, 217
Dusenbury, L., 79, 217

Elders, M. J., 82, 162, 169, 217
Elias, M. J., 33, 217

Elliott, S. N., 204
Emery, R. E., 34, 217
Ennett, S. T., 86, 217
Epstein, J. L., 69, 70, 217
Ershoff, D. H., 89, 178, 179, 217
Evertson, C. M., 68, 217, 218

Falco, M., 196, 218
Fantuzzo, J. W., 63, 73, 218
Farley, C., 121, 122, 218
Fawcett, S. B., 172, 173, 218
Feighery, E., 169, 170, 171, 218
Felner, R. D., 36, 37, 42, 195, 205, 218
Fetterman, D., 197, 218
Finkelhor, D., 38, 137, 138, 218
Finney, J. W., 118, 218
Flay, B. R., 197, 218
Floyd, R. L., 88, 218
Flynn B. C., 196, 219
Flynn, B. S., 77, 78, 79, 219
Forehand, R., 52, 180, 194, 219
Frank, R. G., 157, 219
Franklin, C., 210
Fraser, B. J., 67, 219
Frazier, F., 42, 219
Fullan, M. G., 69, 219
Furstenberg, Jr. F. F., 107, 188, 219

Gardner, W., 107, 219
Gettinger, M., 68, 219
Ginsberg, G. M., 145, 150, 180, 191, 219
Girgis, A., 101, 179, 180, 219
Glenwick, D. S., 205
Gliksman, L., 172, 219
Goldston, S. E., 20, 219
Gramlich, E., 144, 219
Greenberg, R. A., 90, 219
Greenwood, C. R., 63, 64, 180, 219

Grossman, M., 162, 163, 169, 220
Gullotta, T. P., 181, 220

Hamblin, R. L., 21, 220
Hansen, W. B., 77, 78, 85, 178, 179, 220
Harbeck-Weber, C., 35, 220
Hardy, J. B., 135, 220
Hawkins, J. D., 7, 13, 39, 68, 73, 83, 178, 179, 220
Heller, K., 23, 220
Henggeler, S. W., 10, 220
Hetznecker, W., 18, 19, 220
Hobfoll, S. E., 109, 110, 111, 220
Horacek, H. J., 60, 220
Horn, M., 19, 20, 220
Hu, T., 162, 220

Infant Health and Development Program, 91, 186, 220
Institute of Medicine, 13, 23, 196, 205, 220

Jason, L. A., 6, 23, 33, 34, 73, 168, 220, 221
Johnson, C. A., 78, 80, 178, 179, 221
Johnson, D. L., 41, 42, 221
Johnston, L. D., 75, 221
Julnes, G., 98, 221
Jumper, S. A., 131, 221

Kagitcibasi, C., 61, 221
Kaiserman, M. J., 162, 221
Kaplan, R. M., 98, 221
Kaufman, J., 132, 221
Kazdin, A. E., 27, 47, 221
Kelder, S. H., 80, 100, 103, 178, 79, 221
Kellam, S. G., 30, 31, 221
Kelly, J. A., 107, 221
Kendall-Tackett, K. A., 131, 221
Kent, M. W., 206
Kessler, M., 205
Kim, S., 156, 222

King, J. A., 151, 153, 222
Kirby, D., 107, 222
Klein, D. C., 180, 222
Klepp, K. I., 80, 222
Klitzner, M., 22, 222
Knoff, H. M., 70, 73, 178, 186, 222
Knitzer, J., 27, 222
Kohl, J., 23, 137, 138, 222
Kronenfeld, J. J., 160, 222

Ladd, G. W., 204
Lamb, H. R., 9, 222
Lavelle, J. M., 170, 171, 222
Lavigne, J. V., 88, 115, 222
Leigh, B. C., 75, 222
Lev, M. A., 38, 222
Lewit, E. M., 175, 222
Levine, M., 4, 222
Levit, K. R., 62, 199
Lipsey, M. W., 28, 144, 145, 148, 149, 150, 222
Lloyd, J. W., 56, 223
Lochman, J. E., 45, 49, 51, 223
Lombard, D., 100, 101, 102, 223
Long, B. B., 18, 223
Lorion, R. P., 45, 223
Luepker, R. V., 105, 223
Lutzker, J. R., 139, 223

Mac Iver, D. J., 56, 223
MacMillan, H. L., 134, 137, 138, 223
Malinosky-Rummell, R., 131, 223
Manning, W. G., 144, 155, 161, 223
Mayer, G. R., 39, 40, 223
McGrath, M. P., 137, 223
McLeroy, K. R., 159, 223
McMahon, R. J., 52, 223
Mechanic, D., 160, 224
Meehan, M. P., 191, 224
Melamed, B.G., 36, 224
Melton, G. B., 137, 138, 224
Meyer, L. A., 66, 224

Miller, T. R., 115, 144, 145, 146, 180, 224
Morrison, F. J., 62, 224
Morrow, R. H., 146, 224
Moser, Jr., R., 199, 224
Murphy, J., 55, 224

National Academy of Sciences, 116, 224
National Committee for Injury Prevention and Control, 116, 224
National Commission on Children, 76, 224
National Institute of Education, 39, 224
National Safety Council, 117, 224
Nolin, M. J., 38, 224
Nottelmann, E. D., 27, 224

Oakland, T., 200, 224
Oates, R. K., 132, 224
Oden, S., 45, 48, 224
O'Donnell, J., 39, 224
Office of the Inspector General, 168, 225
Ojemann, R.H., 31, 225
Olds, D. L., 91, 95, 134, 135, 145, 157, 179, 186, 225
Olweus, D., 37, 38, 225
O'Malley, P. M., 165, 166, 179, 180, 225
O'Sullivan, A. L., 91, 94, 97, 225

Palumbo, D. J., 160, 225
Pedro-Carroll, J. L., 34, 225
Pentz, M. A., 160, 225
Pendergrast, R. A., 122, 225
Perry, C. L., 77, 78, 80, 100, 102, 103, 171, 178, 179, 191, 225
Perry, M. J., 211
Peterson, D. E., 161, 225
Peterson, L., 36, 118, 128, 133, 226

Philliber, S., 111, 112, 195, 226
Pless, I. B., 122, 226
Preusser, D. F., 169, 226
Price, R. H., 2, 205, 226

Randolph, M. K., 140, 226
Ramey, C. T., 93, 226
Reppucci, N. D., 137, 226
Resnicow, K., 98, 226
Richardson, T. R., 19, 20, 226
Rice, D. P., 157, 226
Rickel, A. U., 45, 48, 49, 226
Riessman, F., 190, 226
Rigotti, N. A., 163, 226
Rivara, F. P., 116, 227
Roberts, M. C., 118, 119, 120, 127, 206, 227
Robertson, L. S., 118, 227
Rodriguez, J. G., 115, 227
Rogers, M. M., 157, 227
Ross, G. R., 31, 227
Ross, J. G., 161, 227
Ross, S., 106, 227
Rotheram-Borus, M. J., 109, 110, 227
Rowan, B., 174, 227
Russell, L. B., 157, 227
Rutter, M., 11, 227

Sameroff, A. J., 4, 9, 11, 227
Samet, J. M., 90, 227
Sandler, I. N., 30, 227
Sarason, S. B., 69, 227
Schelp, L., 123, 124, 125, 178, 179, 228
Schinke, S. P., 76, 192, 227
Schwartz, D. F., 124, 125, 178, 179, 228
Schweinhart, L. J., 59, 193, 228
Simmons, S. J., 23, 228
Simons-Morton, B. G., 100, 103, 104, 178, 179, 228
Seekins, T., 119, 228
Skretny, M. T., 168, 228
Slavin, R. E., 21, 22, 59, 63, 64, 65, 206, 228

Smith, G. S., 118, 228
Snortum, J. R., 164, 228
Soriano, M., 28, 228
Spaulding, J., 18, 228
Spiegel, C. N., 123, 124, 179, 180, 228
Spivack, G., 32, 229
Stephens, T. M., 204
Stevens, R. J., 71, 73, 186, 229
Stevenson, H. W., 72, 229
St. Lawrence, J. S., 109, 110, 178, 179, 229
Stolberg, A. L., 35, 229
St. Pierre, T. L., 79, 195, 229
Sylva, K., 58, 68, 229

Terman, D. L., 55, 174, 229
Tengs, T. O., 147, 229
Thompson, R. S., 121, 229
Tremblay, R. E., 45, 51, 229
Trickett, E. J., 207, 229
Tyack, D., 18, 229

United States Department of Education, 55, 229
United States Department of Health and Human Services, 85, 229
United States Preventive Services Task Force, 129, 229
van den Boom, D. C., 32, 42, 190, 229

Vartiainen, E., 77, 78, 81, 82, 83, 230
Vaux, A., 191, 230
Vegega, M. E., 76, 230
Vinokur, A., 151

Wagenaar, A. C., 164, 169, 230
Walberg, H. J., 56, 230
Wall, M. A., 90, 230
Wallack, L., 198, 230
Walton, W. W., 118, 179, 180, 230
Wasserman, J., 164, 230

Weisbrod, B. A., 143, 230
Wesch, D., 139, 230
Weisz, J. R., 9, 230
Widom, C. S., 132, 230
Williams, S., 167, 230
Williams, A. F., 11, 230
Willis, D. J., 131, 230
Wilson, M. H., 115, 116, 117, 230
Windsor, R. A., 89, 144, 145, 147, 180

Winett, R. A., 198, 206, 230
Wolf, M. M., 156, 230
Wolfe, D. A., 132, 136, 137, 231
Wolfson, M., 165, 231
Wood, T., 121, 231
Writing Group for the DISC Collaborative Research Group, 100, 106, 231

Yap, J. N., 35, 231
Yates, B. T., 144, 231
Yeaton, W. H., 127, 231
Yoshikawa, H., 60, 73, 231

Zabin, L. S., 109, 112, 178, 231
Zimmerman, S. L., 160, 231
Zingraff, M. T., 12, 231

Subject Index

Abecadarian Project, 60; *see also* Early childhood programs
Affective education, 31
Alcohol
  and contracpetive use, 75
  and drunk-driving legislation, 164–165; *see also* Legislation
  and driving fatalities, 76
  and external benefits of prevention, 155
  interventions to prevent use of, 76–83t
  and sales to minors, 169–170
AIDS; *see also* Physical Health
  interventions to prevent, 109–111t
  and risks, 107

Behavioral/social problems
  bullying, 37–39
  crime and violence, 28
  early screening of, 43–44
  extent of, 27–28
  indicated (secondary) prevention of, 43–53f,t
  and preschool children, 48, 52–53
  primary prevention of, 28–42f
  vandalism, 39–40
Bibliographies, on prevention, 207
Bicycle helmets, *see also* Injuries; Legislation
  importance of, 121
  interventions to promote wearing of, 121–126
  and laws, 121–122
Bullying: *see* Behavioral/social problems

Cardiovascular health: *see* Physical health
Child abuse: *see* Maltreatment
Child and Adolescent Trial for Cardiovascular Health (CATCH), 105
Children of Divorce Intervention Project (CODIP), 34–35
Child safety seats, *see also* Injuries; Legislation
  importance of, 118
  interventions to promote use of, 119–120f
Class of 1989 Study, 80, 103; *see also* Drug use; Physical health
Classroom environments, 67–68; *see also* Learning problems
Classwide Peer Tutoring (CWPT), 63–64
Clearinghouses, on prevention, 208–210
Community coalitions
  general importance of, 196–197
  and injury prevention, 121–126t
Community Mental Health Center (CMHC), 19–20
Cost analysis
  benefit–cost analysis, 144
  benefit–cost ratio, 144
  cautions about, 157–158
  consumer reactions in, 156
  cost effectiveness analysis, 150–153t
  distributional effects (equity) of interventions, 154
  external benefits, 155–156
  of bicycle helmet laws, 150
  of child and maternal health programs, 148

Cost analysis (*cont.*)
  of child safety seat program, 120
  of delinquency prevention, 148–150*t*
  of drug prevention, 156
  of early childhood programs, 147–148
  personal benefits, 145–147
  results of, 180*t*
  stakeholder perspectives, 154–155
  time as a program cost, 151–152
CWPT: *see* Classwide Peer Tutoring

Developmental pathways, *see also* Prevention, research and practice, themes in
  and academic problems 14–16*f*
  and adolescence, 14–15*f*
  definitions of, 13
  and life transitions 16*f*
Dietary Intervention Study in Children (DISC), 105–106
DISTAR, 66
Divorce Adjustment Program (DAP), 35
Drug use (substance use)
  current interventions, 77–83*t*
  extent of, 75,
  history of interventions, 76–77

Early childhood programs
  elements of successful interventions, 61–62
  examples of, 59–61*f*
Effective schools
  characteristics of, 68–69
  increasing effectiveness, examples of, 70–72

Food Service, school, changes in, 104–105

Gateway drugs, 85
Good Behavior Game, 30–31
Go For Health Program, 103–104

Head Start, 57–58; *see also* Early childhood programs
Health, general model for 186–188*f*
Health education: *see* Physical health
Health Promotion: *see* Prevention, research and practice, themes in
Healthy Cities, 196; *see also* Community coalitions
Home Team, 102–103

Home visiting
  examples of, 91–92*t*
  value of, 97–98
Houston Parent–Child Development Center, 41

Indicated preventive intervention (indicated prevention): *see* Prevention, general approaches to, definitions of
Implementation
  as aspect of social (public) policy, 160, 167–170
  definition of, 194
  importance of, 194
  of child safety seat legislation, 170–171
  outcomes related to, 194
  strategies to enhance, 194
Infant Health and Development Program (IHDP), 93–94
Informational (educational) programs
  abandon use of, 192–193
  and drug use, 76
  and hospital preparation programs, 35–36
  ineffectiveness of, in general, 192
  and injury prevention, 122–123
Injuries, *see also* Bicycle helmets; Child safety seats
  consequences of, 115
  elements of effective interventions, 126–127
  extent of, 115
  and legislation, 118–119, 121–122
  interventions to prevent, 119–129*f,t*
  and physicians, 129
  risks at different ages, 116–117*t*
International prevention research
  countries represented, 24
  early childhood programs, 61
Interpersonal problem-solving, 31–32

Journals
  publishing on prevention, 207
  special issues (sections) devoted to prevention, 208

Latch-key children, 128–129
Learning problems, *see also* Classroom environments; Effective schools
  early childhood programs 57–63*f*

Learning problems (*cont.*)
  early intervention, importance of, 57
  elements of effective interventions, 66–67
  extent of, 55–56
  factors affecting, 56
  indicated (secondary) prevention of, 65–66
  primary prevention of, 63–65
  and risk factors, 57
  tutoring, 57
Legislation, *see also* Public (social) policy
  as component of public health approach, 163
  Clean Air (no-smoking) Laws, 163–164
  drafting of, 171
  and drug use, 163
  drunk-driving laws, 164–165
  Education Consolidation and Improvement Act, 174
  Education for All Handicapped Children Act, 173
  effects of, in general, 163–167
  enforcement of, 164–165
  and injury prevention, 118–119
  minimum age laws, 165–167f
Life Skills Training (LST), 77–79

Maltreatment
  extent of, 131
  consequences of, 131–32
  intergenerational character of, 132
  physical abuse and neglect
    interventions to prevent, 134–136
    risk and protective factors for, 132–134t
  sexual abuse
    general program procedures, 137
    interventions to prevent, 137–139
    indicated (secondary) prevention of, 139–140
Mass media
  and antismoking campaigns, 162n
  and drug prevention, 79
  effective campaigns, 197
  media advocacy, 197–198
Midwestern Prevention Project, 80
Minnesota Heart Health Project (MHHP), 80; *see* Class of 1989 Study
Mothers Against Drunk Driving (MADD), 174

Multiple causality: *see* Prevention, research and practice, themes in

National Mental Health Association (NMHA)
  aims of, 18
  Beers' contribution to, 18
  and child guidance clinics, 18–19
North Karelia Youth Project (NKYP), 81–82
Nutrition: *see* Physical health

Parents:
  educational practices and attitudes, 72–73
  first-time, interventions for, 32–33
  importance of, in prevention, 192
  involvement and children's academic achievement, 69–70
  training, to prevent behavioral/social problems, 41–42
Perry Preschool Program (PPP), *see also* Early childhood programs,
  cost effectiveness of, 147–148
  outcomes of, 59–60
Physical health, *see also* Smoking
  extent of problems, 87–88
  guidelines for early health intervention, 94–98t
  programs for pregnant women and young children, 88–94
  programs for school-age children, 98–106
  programs for junior high and high school students, 106–113t
Poison Prevention Packaging Act, 118
Positive factors, 10n; *see also* Protective factors
Pregnancy
  extent of, in adolescence, 107
  features of effective programs, 107–108
  interventions, 109t, 111–113
Prevention, general approaches to
  critical questions in, 7–8t
  definitions of,
    primary (selective preventive interventions), 1–2
    secondary (indicated preventive interventions), 1–2
    tertiary, 1–2
  levels of intervention, 3–6f

Prevention, general approaches to (*cont.*)
    target populations, selection of, 2–3*f*
    transition (milestone) programs
        children of divorce, 34–35
        dental and medical treatment, 35–36
        first-time mothers, 32–33
        school entry and change, 33–34
    universal interventions, 2
Prevention, research and practice in,
    collaboration, value of, 195–196, 199
    and community-based organizations, 195
    current status of, 177–181
    disciplines participating in, 1
    extent of current practice, 21–23
    extent of current research, 21–22*f*
    flexibility, need for, 193–194
    for behavioral and social problems, 27–53
    for drug (substance) use, 75–86
    for injuries, 115–130
    for learning problems, 55–74
    for maltreatment, 131–141
    for multiple problems, 186
    for physical health problems, 87–113
    goals of, 6–7
    guidelines, for future, 181–201
    and health care spending, 199
    history of, 17–20
    long-term perspective, needed in, 147–148, 193
    outcomes for, in general, 177–180
    practical benefits of, 178–180*t*
    protective factors in, 188–192*t*
    qualitative approaches in, 198
    sites for, 195
    and social policy, 175
    themes in
        developmental pathways, 13–17*f*
        health promotion, 12–13
        multiple causality, 9–10*f*
        risk and protective factors, 10–12
        skill training, 17
    training and, 199–200
Primary Mental Health Project (PMHP), 44–45
Proactive Classroom Management, 67–68; *see also* Classroom environments
Progressive era, 18

Project Achieve, 70–71
Project DARE, 85–86
Project Northland, 80–81
Project 12-Ways, 139–140
Protective factors, *see also* Risk factors, Positive factors
    and academic performance, 73, 190
    common factors across programs, 189*t*
    definition of, 10
    and parent–child relationship, 190
    and peer modeling and reinforcement, 190
    and social norms, 191
    and social support, 191
Public (social) policy
    bottom-up approaches to influencing, 173–174
    components of, 160
    definition of, 159
    national policy on prevention, 175
    top-down approaches to influencing, 172–175
    and schools, 160–161
Public Service Announcements (PSAs), 197

Quality-of-Life measures, 146

Reciprocal peer tutoring (RPT), 63
Refrigerator Safety Act, 118
Refusal skills: *see* Resistance skills
Resistance skills, 77–79*t*
Resources, on prevention: *see* Bibliographies; Clearinghouses; Journals; Texts; Web pages
Risk factors, *see also* Protective factors, common to multiple problems, 181–184*t*
    definition of, 10
    and maltreatment, 132–134*t*

Safe Block Project (SBP), 125–126
Safe Kids/Healthy Neighborhoods Project (SKHN), 125
Safety skills, 127–129
School Health Education Evaluation (SHEE), 99–100
School Readiness, 62–63; *see also* Early childhood programs
School Transitions Project (STP), 33–34

School Transitions Environment Project (STEP), 36–37
Secondary prevention: *see* Prevention, general approaches to, definitions of
Selective preventive intervention: *see* Prevention, general approaches to, definitions of
Self Center, 112–113
Sexual abuse: *see* Maltreatment
Sex education
    elements of effective programs, 107–108
    interventions, 109–11*t*
    political factors affecting, 106–107
Skill training, *see also* Prevention, research and practice, themes in
    and AIDS prevention, 110–111
    as a protective factor, 188–189*t*
    and drug prevention, 77–79*t*
    of parents, to prevent behavioral/social problems, 41–42
    and physical health promotion, 108
    steps in successful training, 203–204
Skin cancer, 101–102
Smoking
    cigarette sales to minors, 168–170*f*
    during pregnancy, 88–89
    impact on physical health, 84–85
    interventions to prevent, 77–83*f,t*, 89

Smoking (*cont.*)
    passive smoking (second-hand smoke), 89–90
    and school policies, 160–161
Social Development Program (SDP), 39
Social Skills Development Program (SSDP), 49–50*f*
Social support, as a protective factor, 189*t*, 191–192
Success For All (SFA), 64–65

Taxation
    as aspect of social policy, 159
    of alcoholic products, 162–163
    of tobacco products, 161–162
Teachers
    burnout, 69
    involvement in sex abuse prevention, 138, 140
    and staff development, 69
Teen Outreach, 111–112
Texts, recommended, on prevention, 205–206
Training, *see also* Skill training
    and careers in prevention, 211
    importance of, 199–200
Tutoring: *see* Learning problems
Yale–New Haven Project, 71

Web pages, on prevention, 206–207, 211